Dr Newton trained at Kings College Hospital, London and
then completed a general practice vocational training scheme
in Humberside. Following this experience in family practice
he moved back into hospital general paediatrics and developed a specific interest in child and adolescent neurology.
Following higher specialist training he was appointed as
Consultant Paediatric Neurologist to the Children's Hospital
in Manchester in 1983. He has been Director of Clinical
Services at Royal Manchester Children's Hospital since Janu-
ary 1988. His doctoral thesis was written on aspects of the
scope for intervention in pregnancy to prevent low birth-
weight and reduce the incidence of cerebral palsy. He has a
son with Down's syndrome and has been a member of the
Down's Syndrome Association since 1985.

THE
Down's Syndrome
HANDBOOK

A practical guide
for parents and carers

Dr Richard Newton
MD FRCP MRCGP DCH DRCOG

*Written in conjunction with
the Down's Syndrome Association*

Illustrated by
Jennie Smith

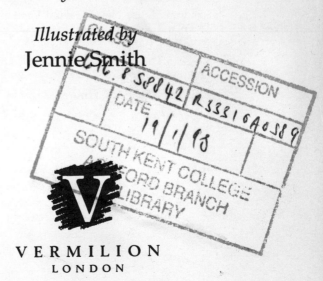
VERMILION
LONDON

First published in the United Kingdom in 1992 by Optima

1 3 5 7 9 10 8 6 4 2

Copyright © Richard Newton and the Down's Syndrome
Association

This edition published in the United Kingdom in 1997 by
Vermilion an imprint of Ebury Press

Random House UK Ltd
Random House
20 Vauxhall Bridge Road
London SW1V 2SA

Random House Australia (Pty) Ltd
20 Alfred Street, Milsons Point, Sydney,
New South Wales 2061, Australia

Random House New Zealand Limited
18 Poland Rd, Glenfield,
Auckland 10, New Zealand

Random House, South Africa (Pty) Limited
Endulini, 5a Jubilee Road, Parktown 2193, South Africa

Random House UK Limited Reg. No. 954009

A CIP catalogue record for this book is available from the
British Library.

ISBN 0 09 181509 6

Typeset in Palatino by Deltatype Ltd, Birkenhead, Merseyside
Printed and bound in Great Britain by Mackays of Chatham, plc

Papers used by Vermilion are natural, recyclable products
made from wood grown in sustainable forests.

CONTENTS

To Judith, Sarah, Michael and Jennifer
as part payment for the time I should have spent
with them whilst writing this text.
And *to the*
DOWN'S SYNDROME ASSOCIATION
for their continuing help and encouragement of
PEOPLE WITH SPECIAL NEEDS

ACKNOWLEDGMENTS

A number of people need appreciative thanks for their contribution to this work. The project was the idea of Sue Brooks, past-director of the Down's Syndrome Association, and she made a major contribution to the text. Elizabeth Blackwell of the South East branch of the DSA wrote some of the section on 'Help with the Baby'; and Shirley Quemby and Jean Shergold of the DSA Education committee made a contribution incorporated in the section on 'Progress at School'.

Daphne Jones, past-Chairman, Roy Dorey, past Director and Anna Khan, immediate-past Director of the DSA, made very useful criticisms and suggestions for which I am grateful. Thanks are also due to Margaret Cunnah for typing the manuscript.

For photographic material I am grateful to David Barker and Rosemary Stevens, young residents at the Home Farm Trust; to Mrs Bryan and Mrs Wadeson of Gaskell Street County Primary School, Bolton and to John Bateman of the department of Medical Illustration, Royal Manchester Children's Hospital.

Finally, I should like to thank Cliff Cunningham and his team and scientists everywhere who through painstaking work have helped establish the facts about Down's syndrome and dispense with the unhelpful myths.

PREFACE

This book has been written to complement existing introductory texts on Down's syndrome, by exploring in more detail many of the common questions raised by parents. In so doing it will clearly be of use not only to parents, family members, teachers and social workers, but also to doctors, health workers and medical students.

Our intention is not to provide an exhaustive supply of specialised information but rather to provide up-to-date general information and, more importantly, practical help and advice. It is hoped that this will assist each person in their attempt to provide a positive environment in which babies, children and adults with Down's syndrome can flourish and reach their full potential.

The majority of people who read this book may only have the opportunity to encounter a small number of people with Down's syndrome. It is the aim of this book to help them make the most of that opportunity.

1

Introduction

'If I could do it then anyone could.' The words of Peter Wiseman, aged 35, having completed his first parachute jump; nothing particularly remarkable about this perhaps, except that Peter has Down's syndrome.

'I would like to be called by my name, not by what's wrong with me.' A plea from Anya Souza, who also has Down's syndrome, and who is employed at the national office of the Down's Syndrome Association.

Two exceptional people who have one thing in common, namely a genetic condition known as Down's syndrome. However, there the similarity ends. Peter and Anya come from very different backgrounds and upbringing, but both have developed a determination not to be typecast by others as a result of their outward appearance or by the label of this particular form of mental handicap. Compared with many children and adults with Down's syndrome, Peter and Anya are high achievers. This has come about through hard work and the support and encouragement of families and enlightened professionals. They have set an example which many could follow.

Down's syndrome is not a disease: it is a genetic condition affecting 800 to 1,000 live births each year in the UK. Children and adults diagnosed as having Down's syndrome are not sufferers or victims; they happen to share some physical characteristics, and also have a degree of learning disability, which varies from person to person. It is important always to remember that, however similar babies and children may look at first glance, they carry family likenesses that become obvious quite quickly. It is also important to remember that physical characteristics are no indication of future ability or capacity to learn, unless there is evidence of life-threatening illness.

Attitudes to people with Down's syndrome have changed over the years, but many of the old prejudices and myths remain. In the rural communities of an earlier age such differences were manageable, but as times changed so did people's attitudes, and little differentiation was made between people who were 'mad', merely 'different' in some way, or just plain 'bad'. The inmates at Bedlam – the Bethlehem Royal Hospital, and the first asylum for the insane in England – and other asylums, were put on show as curiosities. Those with less extreme forms of visible difference were locked away in large institutions, often in the most beautiful country settings, to save them from doing harm to themselves or to others. With very few other resources, and little knowledge about their potential, people were cared for, to a greater or lesser degree for many years, miles away from home and community.

People with Down's syndrome were no exception to this general attitude, but it was not until the middle of the last century that Dr Langdon Down first identified a group of people in an institution and gave the collection of characteristics he had observed an identity. At this time the Victorian medical world had discovered the science of classification. Dr Down, working with the scientific beliefs of the era, concluded that this group of people was a sub-species of the human race, a throwback to 'inferior' non-European races.

Down coined the term 'Mongolian idiots'; variations he called 'negroid idiots', 'Aztec idiots' and 'Malaysian idiots', but none of these latter terms entered the language. Unfortunately the term 'mongol' has become an entrenched part of our language, conjuring up an image of institutional care.

Nowadays people with Down's syndrome, their parents and family, and the professionals who look after them, are sensitive to such outdated images, and do not use the term 'mongol' any more. While it may seem like splitting hairs to talk about terminology, such labels can have a profound effect on the way parents, especially new parents, come to terms with their difficult situation. Furthermore, the word 'mongol' is offensive to people with Down's syndrome, and as an actual description is inaccurate and meaningless.

In the 1950s there was a breakthrough when Professor Lejeune in France discovered that the features that made Down's syndrome so distinctive were genetic in origin. In discovering that an extra chromosome caused Down's syndrome, he started a process of understanding that has given people with Down's syndrome the chance to show what can be achieved, despite their inherent learning difficulties and the disadvantage of others' ignorance.

This change in attitude has in turn brought about a change in opportunity. It is no longer assumed by parents and professionals that babies and children with Down's syndrome should only have basic care, love and attention. From the very first days the children are expected to form as important a part of their family as any other child, with many new parents eager to do something constructive to help give their child the best possible start. Stimulation through loving play, guided by the advice of doctors and therapists, helps parents to focus on a positive way ahead, as well as encouraging early development.

Although the level of ability varies from child to child, many parents aim for integrated activities within the local community. Once children have passed the early crucial years it is possible for them to make great strides into further education and employment. We do not yet know what proportion of men and women with Down's syndrome will live fully independent integrated lives, because it is only since the mid-1970s that so many different opportunities have been given to them. As the present average lifespan of a person with Down's syndrome is about 55 years, we may yet see many more individuals participating much more fully as ordinary members of the community.

2

What is Down's syndrome?

In 1866 Langdon Down first described the characteristics of the commonest recognisable form of mental handicap in Britain. In 1959, 93 years later, Lejeune showed that Down's syndrome was due to extra genetic material carried on chromosome 21 and since that time it has been shown the characteristics of Down's syndrome are due to a relatively small part of the long arm of chromosome 21, (21q22.1–21q22.3, representing perhaps only 50 to 100 genes – see below).

Since 1866 theories on the causation of Down's syndrome and the mechanism of handicap have altered radically. In the 19th century, when Down was alive, it was thought the foetus went through developmental stages in which it assumed different racial characteristics. The legacy of the theory remains, and as recently as 1978 a book was published with the sub-title *The Psychology of Mongolism*. In the same year as Lejeune identified trisomy 21, a paper appeared relating the incidence of Down's syndrome to increased levels of stress in pregnancy. Now Down's syndrome has replaced the term mongolism in scientific literature, and better understanding has allowed us to dispense with spurious beliefs about causation.

It is still not fully known what predisposes dividing cells to retain extra chromosomal material; how this extra material disrupts normal development; nor how function is disrupted as a result. This chapter will summarise the current state of knowledge on these issues and serve to emphasise how much there is yet to be known.

Human genetics

First it is useful to outline some of the basic facts about human genetics.

One of the most exciting developments of the 20th century has been the identification of DNA (deoxyribonucleic acid) as being one of the secrets of life itself. DNA is composed of nucleic acids linked with sugars, capable of forming very long chains and has the further very important property of being able to reproduce and replicate itself. It appears in human cells as a double-stranded helix (spiral); two strands of the spiralled ladder being connected by struts of chemicals called purines and pyrimidines. The two purines involved are called adenine and thymidine, whilst the two pyrimidines are known as cytosine and guanine. The sequence of these basepairs on the DNA molecule is very important in governing cell activity, for it is this sequence that gives the instructing code for which proteins are going to be produced within the cell. Some sections on the DNA molecule code for proteins involved in the structure of the cell; other sections code for proteins known as enzymes, which regulate the activity of chemical reactions within the cell. Any disruption of the structure of DNA would clearly lead to a disruption of either cell structure or cell function, or both.

Most DNA within a human cell is concentrated in the cell nucleus, which often looks denser under the microscope than the rest of the cell contents. Within the cell nucleus the DNA strands are divided up into very small structures called chromosomes. In humans there are 23 pairs of chromosomes, 22 of which are identical, while the 23rd or separate pair (referred to as an X or Y chromosome) determines the sex of an individual. The chromosomes vary in size, with the larger chromosomes governing more activity within the cell than the smaller ones.

Each chromosome is made up of two strands of DNA, each referred to as a chromatid. The chromatids are joined together by chiasmata, which are strands of non-genetic material. Along part of the length of the chromosome the chromatids are very obviously joined together at a specific site known as the centromere. This is usually not in the centre, which means that each chromatid has a long arm and a short arm. The short arm of a chromosome is referred to as p, whilst the long arm is referred to as q. With the special staining technique known as banding, the chromosomes can be divided up into segments. Smaller segments on the DNA molecule which code for

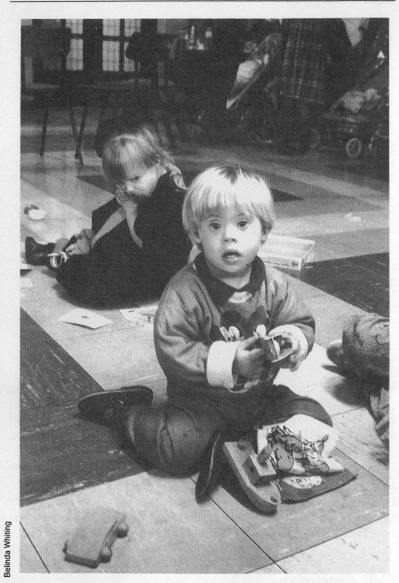

Belinda Whiting

Down's syndrome is not a disease; it is a genetic condition. Children with Down's syndrome are not sufferers or victims, they are people with special, additional needs.

Human Chromosomes from a normal female cell – 23 pairs and two X (female) chromosomes.

particular proteins are known as genes. The extra chromosomal material that leads to the features of Down's syndrome is found on chromosome 21, between segments 21q22.1 and 22.3. This means that the chromosomal material is found between the first and third parts of the 22nd segment on the long arm of the chromosome 21. This small portion of the whole human genome accounts for perhaps only 50 to 100 genes, the function of only a few of which has been identified to date.

Cell division

Somatic division or mitosis

Cells in every tissue in the body are constantly being produced and then die off. This production of cells involves an individual cell line dividing and then dividing again to

Chromosome: low magnification

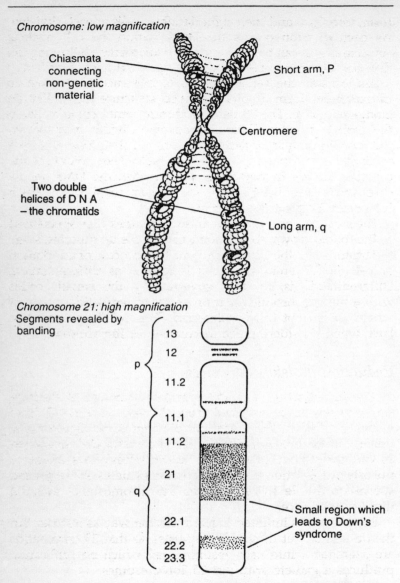

Chiasmata connecting non-genetic material

Short arm, P

Centromere

Two double helices of D N A – the chromatids

Long arm, q

Chromosome 21: high magnification
Segments revealed by banding

13
12
p
11.2
11.1
11.2
21
q
22.1
22.2
23.3

Small region which leads to Down's syndrome

Diagram of chromosome 21 at high magnification. The different segments are revealed by a technique known as banding form, two, four and then eight daughter cells at each division. As each division occurs the DNA within the cell nucleus condenses and can be seen under the microscope, allowing the different chromosomes to be photographed and identified.

Just outside the cell nucleus protein structures known as microtubules form a spindle-shaped structure rather like an elongated globe. The 23 pairs of chromosomes come to lie on the globe's equator. Each chromosome divides into two so that one chromatid passes to one pole of the globe, with the other chromatid passing to the other pole. The contents of the cell then divide in two along the equator, the DNA in the chromatids reduplicating itself so that each resulting cell has a full set of 23 chromosome pairs.

The structure and function of cells becomes very specialised as the foetus grows, so that some cells make up muscles, some the brain, some the skin and so on. This process of adaptation of cells to different functions is known as differentiation. Differentiation is, in turn, governed by the genetic codes within the cell through strict processes of regulation, many of which we do not fully understand. This will be returned to later when considering the mechanism of impairment.

Reduction division or meiosis

In the formation of eggs and sperm the number of chromosomes needs to be reduced from 23 pairs to just 23. This means that, when the sperm and the egg come together, the first cell of the new individual will have the normal number of 23 pairs restored. In order to achieve this the process of meiosis or reduction division leads the gamete cells (eggs and sperm) to divide twice, whereas the chromosomal material divides only once.

The process is initiated in just the same way as mitosis, but then a second set of spindles appears so that 23 chromatids are segregated into each resulting cell which on replication produces a gamete with just 23 chromosomes.

Disordered division

- *Non-disjunction.* If a cell divides and more chromosomal material goes to one pole than the other, then the daughter cells produced will have an abnormal number of chromo-

23 chromosome
pairs

Chromosomes become visible in nucleus. Spindle begins to form

Nucleus wall breaks up, chromosomes attached to spindle by centromere.

*MITOSIS –
SOMATIC DIVISION*

23 chromotid pairs
to each pole

Each chromosome splits in two – one chromotid to one pole and one to the
other

23 chromosome pairs
restored

The D N A replicates – each chromotid becomes a new daughter
chromosome. A nucleus wall reforms and the cytoplasm splits to give the
complete daughter cells.

The sequence of events in mitosis – somatic division.

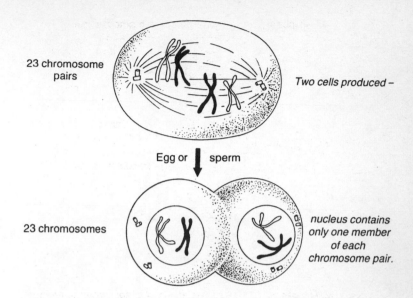

23 chromosome pairs

Two cells produced –

Egg or sperm

23 chromosomes

nucleus contains only one member of each chromosome pair.

Formation of egg and sperm. The first meiotic or reduction division.

somes. This is called aneuploidy; one will show too many chromosomes (hyperploidy) and one too few (hypoploidy). This disordered movement of chromosomes is called non-disjunction and is the commonest cause of the trisomy (three chromosomes rather than the usual pair) that causes Down's syndrome.

- *Translocation.* In the course of cell division it is also possible for a segment of chromosomal material to be attached to another chromosome in an abnormal way. This is known as a translocation of genetic material. If a cell divides to produce a daughter cell with the normal 23 pairs of chromosomes plus a translocation of material from chromosome 21, this will lead to the features of Down's syndrome. On the other hand it is possible, depending on how the chromosomes segregate on the equator of the spindle at cell division, for the translocated material to go to the same pole of the spindle as the chromosome from

Human chromosomes, showing trisomy 21. Note the three chromosomes at the 21 position, instead of the usual two.

which this extra material broke off. In these circumstances one chromosome would be smaller than usual whilst another would carry the extra genetic material. This is known as a balanced translocation and the person is likely to be normal.

- *Mosaicism.* If cell division goes wrong at the stage of early foetal development, but after the first few somatic divisions, then only a few cell lines may be involved in translocation or non-disjunction. In this case examination of different tissues of the body will show that some cells have the normal number of chromosomes whereas others show extra genetic material. This is known as mosaicism.

Disordered division and Down's syndrome

As long as a person carries the extra segment of chromosomal

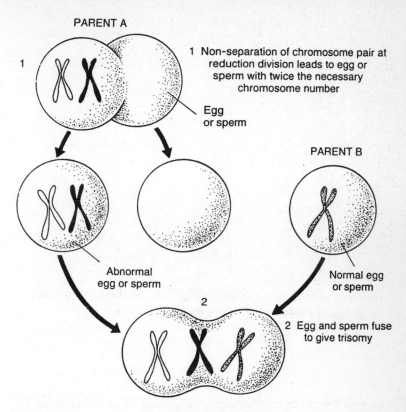

Diagrammatic representation of non-disjunction.

material from chromosome 21 (segments 21q22.1–21q22.3) they will have Down's syndrome, whether it be through a non-disjunction of the chromosomal material or a transloca-tion. The range of abilities therefore are likely to be the same in each group. For people with mosaicism, however, relatively few cell lines can be affected and on the whole this group tend to have relatively less disability. It must be said, however, that there is a huge overlap in the ability of people with Down's syndrome mosaicism and those with other forms of Down's syndrome.

Incidence of Down's syndrome according to maternal age.

Down's syndrome is most commonly due to trisomy 21. The trisomy arises because of a non-disjunction of chromosomes at the reduction division. Trisomy may arise either during the first or the second meiotic division.

About 5 per cent of children with Down's syndrome will have a translocation, the extra chromosome 21 material having attached itself to one of the D group (chromosomes 13, 14 or 15), chromosome number 14 being the commonest. In about 1 per cent of cases the G group chromosomes, numbers 21 or 22, will be involved. Translocations may arise for the first time in the affected child, but chromosomal analysis in the parents may reveal mosaicism or a balanced translocation to be the cause.

Mosaicism is rare and accounts for up to 5 per cent of Down's syndrome.

Risk factors for Down's syndrome

A number of theories have been developed to explain observations on the incident of Down's syndrome. The incidence in women under 20 years of age is less than 1 in 2,000, rising to something like 1 in 20 at the age of 45. The steepest increment in incidence with maternal age occurs at the age of 35, although it must be remembered that half of those mothers who give birth to a child with Down's syndrome are less than 35 years old. In recent years there has been an increasing incidence amongst younger mothers, partly because women are deciding to have their families earlier.

There are clearly factors other than maternal age which are important, increasing paternal age being one of these.

The effect of paternal age on incidence of Down's syndrome		
Paternal age	*Maternal age*	
	35–40 (%)	41–46 (%)
34	0.4	0.8
35–40	0.6	1.2
41–46	1.3	2.8
47	2.0	4.1

After Stene *et al.*, 1981.

Although the impact of paternal age is not as marked as that of maternal age, the effect seems to be derived from the aging of sperm. Animal studies have shown that the longer sperm is stored in the genito-urinary tract, the greater the incidence there is of sperm-derived trisomies. Decreased frequency of sex means that the sperm ejaculated are relatively older. This could be part of the explanation for the increased incidence of Down's syndrome in babies born to older couples, who might be expected to have a decreased frequency of sexual intercourse. It might also explain the increasing number of babies with Down's syndrome born to unmarried teenage couples who, because they do not live together, do not have intercourse as frequently as co-habiting/married couples.

It is possible to determine the parental origin of the extra chromosomal material by studying chromosomal variants (heteromorphisms). A number of studies have reliably shown that in about 80 per cent of trisomies the extra chromosome has its origins in non-disjunction at the first maternal reduction division. There is then no support for the theory that the 'older' eggs of an 'older woman' increase the risk of trisomy; this first meiosis takes place in the ovary long before the mother herself is born.

The remainder of heteromorphisms take their origin in the second maternal meiotic division or in the first or second paternal meiotic divisions. It is known that the crossover of chromosomal material and non-disjunction may be caused by reduced chiasmata formation, the chiasmata being the non-genetic strands that help paired chromosomes adhere to each other. Chiasmata formation occurs before birth in females and reduces with age, making it more likely for genetic material to split off in an abnormal way. Increasing maternal age therefore leads to an increase in the number of cells with an abnormal number of chromosomes.

The development of many abnormal foetuses is arrested by a process called micronucleation or extrusion. Thus, the vast majority of pregnancies involving abnormal foetuses miscarry spontaneously, often at a very early stage. Research is currently focusing on whether there is an increased production of abnormal embryos as the sole cause of the increased frequency with age, or whether there is actually a decrease in this natural process of selective destruction.

Foetuses showing a reduced number of chromosomes (hypoploidy) cannot survive, as the effect on the growing metabolism is too great. Hyperploidy (too many) of the larger chromosomes, with their great effect on body metabolism, also seems to lead to foetal elimination. However, hyperploidy of the smaller chromosomes, with a lesser effect, is often compatible with survival. As chromosome 21 is one of the smallest, Down's syndrome comes to be the commonest recognisable form of mental handicap.

The development of more sophisticated techniques has led to greater insights into the ways in which the reduction division may go wrong. One of these techniques, using DNA probes that recognise specific points on the chromosome, has allowed scientists to map out chromosome 21 and define the point of any chromosomal abnormality. To date, 50 such markers are available, allowing up to 100 per cent accuracy in the prediction of the site and type of abnormality. This technique will doubtlessly improve our future understanding.

The part environmental factors, such as X-rays, chemicals and viruses, may play on some of these chromosomal events is as yet unproven. Hormonal factors may be of importance; an increased frequency of chromosome abnormality has been noted in the pregnancies which miscarry in women of any age who are users of the contraceptive pill. It can readily be seen how male workers in areas of radiation exposure may suffer abnormalities at the first and second paternal meiotic division, as the production of new sperm goes on throughout life.

There also may be inherent biological vulnerability factors in some individuals, outside environmental influence. For example one study showed the cells of mothers of children with Down's syndrome to have a variation of microtubular function, the microtubules forming the spindle on which the separation of the chromosomes takes place at the time of cell division. These observations need to be confirmed by further studies before firm conclusions can be drawn.

Prevention

At present there seems to be little scope for prevention in Down's syndrome. The environmental factors cited above have no more than speculative importance at this stage, although if any were to become better defined, attention to safety standards at work and political influences of an environmental and ecological nature could lead to a reduction in background risk.

Further study may help us identify those with a genetic predisposition, and appropriate counselling could ensue. Meanwhile the only substantive evidence we have is that the incidence of trisomy 21 of paternal origin (20 to 25 per cent of the total) might be reduced by increasing and sustaining coital frequency. This will be encouraging to the more amorous and energetic members of our society!

Characteristics of Down's syndrome

The phenotype refers to the observable features of a genetic condition; it includes physical appearance, behaviour and intellectual function.

Physical appearance

The physical features of Down's syndrome are known to most people, allowing identification of the vast majority in the newborn period. Obvious floppiness (hypotonia) is a striking and consistent feature in all but a few (see photograph overleaf).

It should be remembered that there is a wide range of characteristics; few children exhibit them all, and some only a few. It must be said that in some children the diagnosis can be difficult, and only chromosomal analysis in these cases will exclude or confirm the condition. Modern laboratory techniques allow an answer within 72 hours, although in practice, due to laboratory workload, it often takes longer.

Down's syndrome – phenotype

Hypotonia – Flexible joints
Learning difficulties
Mild microcephaly – brachycephaly
Epicanthic folds – Mongoloid slant – Brushfield spots
Lens opacity – refractive error
Small ears
Dentition – Hypoplasia, irregular placement
         – less caries
Neck – short
Hands – Short metacarpals and phalanges
        – Clinodactyly
        – Simian crease
        – Dermatoglyphics
Feet – gap between first and second toes
Pelvis – hypoplasia – outward lateral flare
Heart – anomolous in 40 per cent
Skin – dry
Hair – sparse
Genitalia – small penis. Low fertility

Newborn infant with Down's syndrome, showing marked floppiness (hypotonia).

The most consistent features in Down's syndrome are the facial appearance, the skeletal structure leading to short stature, and the developmental anomalies of the heart. The importance of the more common characteristics will be re-addressed in the chapter on health issues.

Mental abilities and structure of the brain

Developmental variations are seen in the brain in Down's syndrome. At the macroscopic level (features seen with the naked eye) such variations can be seen in the pathways that are of importance in processing visual information and memory. These include the anterior commisure, which is smaller in Down's syndrome due to underdevelopment. The commisure represents bands of nerve cells which connect different parts of the brain, and particularly the two limbic systems which are involved in memory function.

The brain is a living computer made up of millions of nerve cells, each nerve cell communicating with its neighbour through small outgrowths called dendrites. The quality and

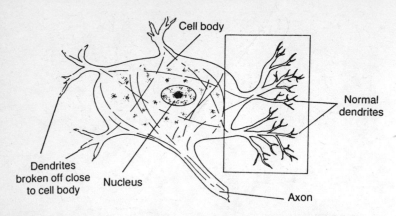

Diagram to show motor nerve cell with the axon (nerve cell body) and dendrites (nerve cell connectors) broken off near to the body of the cell. Two normal dendrites are shown for comparison.

quantity of these dendrites determines the level of computing and learning ability. At the microscopic level abnormal dendritic processes can be seen in Down's syndrome.

These structural variations, and the malfunction that accompanies them, have a general deleterious effect on higher cerebral function. However, impairment of learning ability has been overemphasised in the past, and the full potential for people with Down's syndrome has only been realised since they have had ready access to education and not been committed to an institutional existence. Overall, there is a very broad range of ability within Down's syndrome, from profound learning difficulties to low/average intelligence. Most children with Down's syndrome have mild to moderate learning difficulties.

Emotional, psychological and social stereotypes have been described, but in practice these descriptions do not bear close scrutiny. In general people with Down's syndrome have as many behavioural characteristics as the population as a whole. Comments like 'They love music, don't they?' or 'They are very loving, aren't they?' should not be accepted at face value. These issues will be readdressed in the chapter on growing up and adult life.

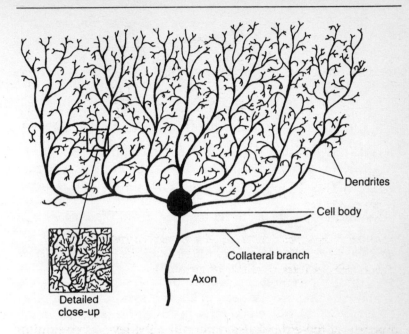

A close-up of a neurone in the cerebellum (one of the motor control cells in the brain), showing the rich network of dendrites normally present and great scope for computing ability!

Mechanism of impairment

Dysembryogenesis (malformation of the foetus)

It is one thing to say extra chromosomal material causes Down's syndrome, but another thing entirely to understand exactly what the mechanism is. It is clear that dysembryogenesis is an important factor affecting many vital organs. But when one considers the complexity of human development, it is surprising that it does not go wrong more often. The process of differentiation of different cell lines and their organisation into different body organs is ordered or buffered by biofeedback mechanisms which are poorly understood.

In Down's syndrome the extra genetic material seems to lead to a disturbance of the controlling mechanisms, which allows developing organs to become disordered. This mechanism has been referred to as amplified developmental instability. This influence can best be understood by considering that 80 per cent of the manifestations of Down's syndrome are actually minor anomalies seen frequently in isolation in other normal people (for example Brushfield spots or epicanthic folds).

Cell dysfunction and metabolic disorder

Normal cell function is highly dependent on the activity of enzymes, an enzyme being a biochemical that helps along an essential body process without itself being altered in structure.

One of the first genes to be mapped on to the long arm of chromosome 21 was that coding for the enzyme superoxide dismutase (SOD-1). This enzyme is important in the generation of a disruptive process known as lipoperoxidation. Because of the central importance of lipoperoxidation in the premature aging process seen in Down's syndrome, and other consequences of cell membrane malfunction (such as faulty neurotransmitter production), it will be dealt with below in some detail.

Other enzyme systems coded on 21q are:

- The production of a protein involved with cataract formation (alpha-A crystal protein) at segment 21q22.
- At 21q21 is an enzyme involved in one stage of glucose production and metabolism (phosfructokinase). Its overactivity may account for a reported excess prevalence of diabetes in people with Down's syndrome.
- An enzyme (cystathionine synthase) that lowers the risk of arteriosclerosis (furred-up arteries), tying in with the fact that people with Down's syndrome have a lower than usual risk of this sort of heart disease.
- Overactive enzyme systems that affect cell membranes appear to be responsible for a number of characteristics, including premature aging. A form of pre-senile dementia called Alzheimer's disease is very common in Down's syndrome. Those genes coding for familial Alzheimer's disease have been shown to lie adjacent to the protein precursors of an important protein in this disease called amyloid (see chapter on medical aspects).

- Cell membranes in the body's defence system may also malfunction, making infection and malignancy more common. The augmented risk of leukaemia may be associated with the presence of a cancer susceptibility gene known as oncogene ets-2 at segment 21q22. A further gene associated with oestrogen-dependent breast cancer (BCEI) lies adjacent, but the significance of this for women with Down's syndrome is not yet clear as there is no reported excess of that disorder.
- Interferon, a protein with strong anti-viral properties, is also coded for on chromosome 21. Although overproduced because of the gene dosage effect (that is, three rather than two genes are present), it seems far less effective.
- The balance of some neurotransmitters – the biochemicals that are responsible for transporting messages around the brain and nervous system – is also affected. The precise effect of this is as yet only poorly understood.

Cell malfunction, lipoperoxidation and premature aging

The proteins produced on chromosomal DNA pass out into the cytoplasm, the fluid that fills cells. Here they join with fat (lipid) molecules such as cholesterol and polyunsaturated fatty acids to form the complex lipoprotein structures that make up cell walls, and the smaller power-houses and production lines within the cell that contribute to cell function. Lipoperoxidation disrupts the structure of these lipoproteins, and allows oxygen-containing chemicals known as free radicals to become attached to them.

The enzyme called superoxide dismutase (SOD-1, see above) has been shown to be 50 per cent more active in people with Down's syndrome. It is responsible for the metabolism of oxygen-free biochemicals and, in so doing, produces oxygen-containing free radicals. It is important that not too many of these free radicals are around in the cell as many vital cellular processes depend on controlled free-radical metabolism. This is particularly true of the energy production that goes on in tiny intra-cellular power-houses called mitochondria; and for the lipid, protein and glucose release that takes place from another structure known as the endoplasmic reticulum.

Excessive free radical production is at least partly controlled by an enzyme called glutathione peroxidase, along with other catalases (which break down rather than build up) and radical scavengers such as alpha-tocopherol (which collect up and neutralise these free radicals). When these are inefficient, then the polyunsaturated fatty acids and cholesterol that make up the lipid membrane on the surface of nerve cells become vulnerable.

An increase in lipoperoxidation could explain some of the premature aging effects seen in Down's syndrome. Pathological studies have shown that, whereas the acquisition of cortical neurones in Down's syndrome is unaffected, the dentritic spines on individual neurones are reduced from the early post-neonatal period onwards. This is due to a premature arrest of growth, so that by the time adult life is reached the dendritic spine deficiency is quite severe. It is through the growth of these dendritic spines that one neurone can communicate with another, thus building up more complex computer circuitry and allowing thought, deduction and learning at a higher level.

Studies have shown that abnormal membrane properties are seen in the peripheral tissues of older people with Down's syndrome, and an abnormality of metabolism seen in normal cellular aging has also been defined. Alzheimer's disease and the high prevalence of cataract are further examples of the analogy that can be drawn between pathological changes in older people with Down's syndrome and what occurs in other humans at a later age.

Any damaging effect of increased SOD-1 activity may be present from early on in foetal life. In the foetal brain it has been shown that SOD-1 activity is increased, with no corresponding increase in the protective effect of glutathione peroxidase activity or alpha-tocopherol, cited above as a free radical scavenger and a major lipid anti-oxidant. Therefore brain cells may be more susceptible at an early age, when compensatory mechanisms do not exist. The polyunsaturated fatty acid profile of cell surface membranes has also been shown to resemble those in the brains of older individuals, though the profiles show that the pattern is distorted rather than being merely advanced in years.

The metabolism of some vitamins and trace elements

Many parents ask about the value of dietary supplements. While considering aspects of metabolism, it is timely to consider vitamins and trace elements (coenzymes), without which enzymes cannot function efficiently. The following two sections will put their importance into perspective.

Folate metabolism

Although the average serum folate and vitamin B12 levels in Down's syndrome appear to be normal, red cell folate levels have been shown to be very low. There is a corresponding increase in the presence of large red blood corpuscles (macrocytosis) and ultimately a lower serum folate level seen with age. Leukaemia-like nuclear ultrastructural abnormalities in the white blood corpuscles (leucocytes) of people with Down's syndrome have also been shown to be tenfold more common than usually found. These nuclear membrane abnormalities do not correlate with serum folate, but both factors are associated with chromosome breakage, which may be partly responsible for the increased risk of malignant change and particularly leukaemia seen in Down's syndrome.

It may thus be of value to monitor red cell folate levels at infrequent intervals, particularly in adult life. If they are shown to be low, folate supplements may be of benefit.

Trace elements

A number of groups have studied trace elements in people with Down's syndrome. One clear message from all these studies is that hair analysis is completely unreliable as a reflection of body metabolism. Many laboratories offer this on a private basis to professionals and parents alike, and they should be avoided.

Glutathione peroxidase is the enzyme, already discussed, that protects against lipo-peroxidation, and it has been shown to need selenium to work efficiently. Early studies had suggested that people with Down's syndrome were plasma selenium deficient. It had been postulated that this leads to a compromise of this protective effect, with a resulting increase in susceptibility to Alzheimer's disease and infection. More recent work has, however, failed to replicate these results and a recent Swedish study has shown that plasma selenium is the same as in other people, with red cell selenium actually being higher and reaching adult levels earlier.

Lipoperoxidation is a process that has been likened to premature aging. A number of features of this are seen in Down's syndrome. Vitamin E has been shown to have a protective effect when free radicals begin to accumulate in a variety of clinical conditions. However, this research has only been related to short term benefit. Vitamin E has not been shown to offer long term benefit in Down's syndrome. On theoretical grounds it can be argued that there would be some benefit from long term administration of Vitamin E. However, the scientific study that would be needed to demonstrate this would be very difficult to construct. This issue is likely to become clearer over the next few years as the complex biochemistry involved is better understood.

Trace elements have also been studied in red cells, white cells and platelets in people with Down's syndrome. Copper levels have been shown to be consistently raised in all three blood cell types, and it is notable that SOD-1 is copper dependent. Calcium has also been shown to be raised in red cells. Reductions have been seen in the concentrations of zinc and manganese in red cells, of manganese in platelets, with slight reductions of manganese and iron in red and white cells. Titanium has been found in increased levels in most people with Down's syndrome; in the population at large it is not usually raised except in patients with acute myeloid leukaemia. Again there may be a relationship here between this observation and susceptibility to certain types of malignancy.

Other than this, no conclusions can be drawn from these experimental findings; rather than showing a deficiency, low levels might actually represent a beneficial protective compensatory mechanism. Clearly further study is required.

Summary and conclusions

Down's syndrome is a result of extra chromosomal material present in 50 to 100 genes on the long arm of chromosome 21. In 95 per cent the cause is trisomy 21, and in about 5 per cent an unbalanced translocation or mosaicism. In 80 per cent of those with trisomy 21 the origin of the extra chromosome is at the time of the first maternal meiosis; that is, in the mother's own foetal life. Genetic factors have been shown to be of importance in relation to vulnerability to non-disjunction at this stage. In the remaining 20 per cent or so the origin is at the stage of maternal meiosis II or paternal meiosis I or II. Reduced chiasmata formation may be important here, as may be the length of time spermatozoa spend in the male genital tract. Environmental agents such as radiation and the contraceptive pill are putative risk factors. Further study is required.

Most of the manifestations of Down's syndrome are minor anomalies seen frequently in isolation in other normal people. The effect of the increased gene dosage seems to decrease the buffering of potential disorder in developmental pathways. The resulting amplified developmental instability leads to a far greater incidence of these minor anomalies. In the brain and the heart this has an important effect on developmental abilities and general health. Furthermore, disordered enzyme activity leads to an enhancement of biochemical processes, and in particular of lipid peroxidation, which mimic many aspects of premature aging. In particular, deleterious effects are seen in relation to neurotransmitter formation and the immune process.

3

Incidence, risk of recurrence and antenatal diagnosis

As discussed earlier, the overall incidence of Down's syndrome is 1:660 new borns. The incidence in women under 20 years of age is less than 1:2,000, rising to something like 1:20 at the age of 45. The steepest increment in incidence according to maternal age occurs after the age of 35.

Risk of recurrence

Parents who have had one child with Down's syndrome may wish to know whether it is possible to have another such child.

Overall risk figures for recurrence are set at about 1 per cent for standard trisomy 21 in women under 35, while after the age of 35 recurrence risk closely parallels that in the age-related population. When either parent carries a balance translocation on either the D group or chromosome 22 the risk of recurrence may be as high as 1:5 where the mother is a carrier, or 1:20 where the father is a carrier. For the very rare 21/21 translocation, all subsequent children will have the condition where either parent is a carrier.

After the birth of any child with Down's syndrome, it is therefore advisable for parents to have genetic counselling, which would usually include the drawing up of a very accurate family tree, examination of the parents and a blood test for chromosomal analysis.

Risk of recurrence of Down's syndrome	
Present baby has	*Risk of recurrence*
Standard trisomy 21	
Parents under 30–35	*1 in 100*
Parents over 35	*Depends on age (see page 28)*
Mosaic trisomy 21 and *Translocation trisomy 21 where a parent is not a carrier* — *Not related to age but so rare that accurate figures are not available*	
Translocation trisomy 21	
D/G translocation (13, 14 or 15/21)	*Between*
When mother is carrier	*1 in 5 and 1 in 10*
When father is carrier	*1 in 20 and 1 in 50*
G/G translocation 21/22	
When mother is carrier	*1 in 5 and 1 in 10*
When father is carrier	*1 in 20 and 1 in 50*
G/G translocation 21/22	
When mother is carrier	*1 in 1*
When father is carrier	*1 in 1*

After Cunningham, C.C., 1988.

Antenatal diagnosis

Amniocentesis

Currently, amniocentesis is offered to most women in Britain aged 35 or over at about 16 weeks' gestation. In amniocentesis a sample of amniotic fluid is obtained and analysed, as it contains foetal cells that can be grown and examined for chromosome abnormality.

The amniocentesis is performed by numbing a small area of skin on the lower abdomen with local anaesthetic, and drawing up the amniotic fluid with a needle and syringe, rather like sampling blood. The risk of miscarriage following amniocentesis is about 1 per cent.

If all women in Britain over 35 had the test, then 7.5 per cnt of pregnancies would require amniocentesis and 35 per cent of cases of Down's syndrome would be detected.

Syringe withdrawing
fluid

Amniotic fluid
surrounding foetus

Bladder

Vagina

Wall of
uterus

Bowel

Diagram of how amniocentesis is performed. A needle is advanced through the lower abdominal wall into the uterus. Fluid and cells are withdrawn from the amniotic sac.

Other biochemical tests

It is also known that Down's syndrome in the foetus is associated with low maternal concentrations of alphafoetoprotein and unconjugated oestriol and a high concentration of human gonadotrophin. A risk factor can be derived from these biochemical tests by relating them to maternal age. This offers a new method of screening, known as the 'triple test', which would allow 60 per cent of affected pregnancies to be detected and the overall amniocentesis rate to be reduced to about 5 per cent. This would potentially reduce the number of children born with Down's syndrome in the United Kingdom from about 900 to 350 a year, if those involved wished to terminate the pregnancy. A further biochemical substance known as neutrophil alkaline phosphatase also allows affected pregnancies to be identified with greater accuracy.

Health commissions in the United Kingdom are currently deciding which method of screening to introduce, their thoughts being centred on cost efficiency and effectiveness. It is essential that all families involved in this screening are offered good counselling on the choices available.

Chorionic villus sampling

A first trimester chorionic villus biopsy offers an alternative method of antenatal diagnosis.

The placenta attaches to the wall of the uterus by little 'fingers' or villi. A probe is inserted via the cervix and one of the villi removed and analysed, giving the same sort of information as is obtained from amniocentesis. Given that currently the quoted risk to the foetus of this test is in the order of 2 to 3 per cent, compared with a 1 per cent risk with amniocentesis, it should probably be reserved for those women with a particularly high risk of recurrence in subsequent pregnancies.

Appropriate counselling should be given before and after both these procedures, and sensitivity will be needed to help with parent's feelings if a positive diagnosis is made, particularly if termination is chosen.

Ultrasound scanning

As the technique of ultrasound scanning has become more sophisticated, so its use has been directed at detecting the presence of Down's syndrome in the developing foetus. For example, if the foetus head can be examined by ultrasound it is possible to identify the characteristic shape. Another technique is to look for a thickened skinfold at the back of the neck, and a femur (thigh bone) that is shorter than would be expected. If these observations are combined with ultrasound detection of heart abnormalities (which are common in Down's syndrome), the technique is about 80 per cent accurate. As it is very time-consuming, the procedure is not widely available; also, it cannot be performed until the foetus

Ultrasound to guide probe

Flexible biopsy tube introduced through vagina and cervix to edge of placenta

Developing foetus

Diagram of how chorionic villus biopsy is performed. A flexible tube is introduced into the vagina through the neck of the womb into the developing chorion. A biopsy is taken.

has developed sufficiently, some time after the 12–14 week stage.

The conclusion is that the use of ultrasound alongside the tissue analysis techniques of amniocentesis and chorionic villus sampling and the biochemical tests such as alphafoeto-protein analysis will allow antenatal diagnosis of Down's syndrome in an ever-growing number of pregnancies, and allow parents concerned an ever greater choice. It must be remembered that these clinical methods will only be of real value to parents when they are accompanied by appropriate counselling. There will always be parents who decide not to involve themselves in these diagnostic methods because they value life for life itself.

4

Hearing the news

To the happy parents of a newborn baby it comes as an enormous surprise or shock to receive the news that their child may have Down's syndrome. Unless an antenatal diagnosis was made they will have had no warning. The surprise can be even greater if the parents are young, because it is still assumed by the lay-public that babies with Down's syndrome are only born to mothers in their late 30s or older. Although the risk is higher for older mothers, half the women who give birth to a baby with Down's syndrome are younger than 35, with many in their 20s and a small number who are in their teens.

Despite the very positive changes in attitudes and knowledge about Down's syndrome, it is regrettable that one of the most painful and traumatic experiences many parents of babies with Down's syndrome remember is the manner in which they were told the news by health care professionals, and the kind of support and follow-up they received.

When asked about this experience many parents wanted the following:

- To be told as soon as possible.
- To be told together.
- To be told sympathetically, in private and with respect for their feelings.
- To have the baby present.
- To be given accurate information.
- To be helped to pass on the news to family and friends.

Tell us as soon as possible

What is invariably meant by this is 'Tell us as soon as everybody else is pretty sure'. If there is any doubt over the diagnosis of Down's syndrome it is important that this possibility is discussed with parents at an early stage.

It is to be expected that parents would wish to be included in such discussions as soon as possible. They may have already sensed that something is not quite right soon after delivery; even if they have not actually recognised the signs in the baby's features, the sense that all is not well can be picked up from the attitude of the maternity staff.

The delivery of simple facts as soon as possible will allow parents to dispense with some of the bad and frightening images they had held previously. This will help them begin to value their baby and realise that they will be able to look after a child with learning difficulties.

Tell us together

The majority of parents want to be told with their partner or close relative present. A relative or friend can often help parents to recall information and reduce their sense of isolation. Sadly, however, it is still the case that most parents can expect to receive the information without this support.

Value the baby

A significant feature of surveys is that parents want their baby to be present with them when they are told of the diagnosis.

Often the baby is not present at this time. This may appear to parents as if the child is not valued, perhaps because of its condition. It is inevitable that parents are sensitive to the attitudes and behaviour of the maternity and medical staff.

Staff need training on how to handle this counselling and to develop their own positive attitude to disability. However, lack of this knowledge should not prevent staff from being friendly, sympathetic and supportive.

Parents should be encouraged to spend as much time as possible with their new baby, and particularly if the baby is on the special care baby unit. When the baby is present staff should react to it as with any other baby by holding, rocking, and talking.

'The baby was in the room but the doctor never looked at it once.'

'The doctor used to come every day, but she never touched

the baby.'

These are two kinds of experience that left parents feeling hurt.

How parents are told is also important. The doctor may not be able to say 'You are very lucky. You have a baby with Down's syndrome', but 'I am terribly sorry, I have some very bad news for you' is too negative. 'I have some news for you which you were not expecting' would be better.

Doctors can also mislead by being too positive. If they propose all kinds of therapy in the wrong light, then parents may think that therapy can 'put the problem right', whereas the real value in the advice therapists give is in encouraging children to reach their full potential (see Chapter 10 for more discussion of this important issue). Doctors should be aware of the values and interpretations that parents attach to such statements, and try to be more factual, balanced and supportive.

Give accurate information and continuing support

In the past parents have often received the news that their child has Down's syndrome in a way that has left them with some anger, confusion or despair. A number of studies over the years have identified the way in which families would prefer to receive the news. Over the last two years SCOPE has established a multidisciplinary working party so that members of the different professions involved might be encouraged to decide on a good standard of practice. This is seen as an important standard and health commissions are being encouraged to incorporate this standard in their contracts with providers delivering the service. The Community Care Act now specifically states that doctors must introduce families to organisations in the voluntary sector likely to give them support and advice. The campaign steered by SCOPE is known as 'Right from the Start'. Its essential ingredients are as follows:

Parents want accurate information. Even when it is available, they may not be able to absorb it when they are so upset, particularly if the doctor only allows one chance to answer questions.

'I didn't have enough time to take it in.'

'I'd have liked to have seen someone else.'

'I needed to talk to somebody afterwards.'

These are all typical comments from parents.

Giving parents enough time and the chance to talk to someone is a long process, and needs to be planned. Ideally the first interview should be short, as parents are so upset in their state of initial shock that they cannot take much in. The doctor giving the news should be experienced and known to them. It is valuable to have another health care professional, such as a health visitor or social worker, present; they will help re-explain what the doctor has said, to enable the parents to gather their thoughts and questions in time for the next interview with the doctor.

This second interview should take place within 24 hours. At this time parents can be introduced to other sources of information, such as parent support groups like the Down's Syndrome Association. Wherever possible simple written information should be provided to complement what has been said by the doctor.

Some parents may need help on how to pass on the information to other family members and friends. Grandparents can be supportive, although initially they may react by saying that the doctors are wrong and that everything will be all right. Siblings may find it hard to tell friends and teachers; family friends may feel helpless and awkward. Parents have found that a simple and honest approach works best. Health visitors can help by talking to family and friends, but most parents prefer to do it themselves. Some typical experiences are:

When telling relatives and friends that our much-wanted first child had Down's syndrome we knew that they would find the news sad, and so we broke it gently. Subsequently our son has been accepted and visited by all.

I am a great believer in being direct with people and not beating about the bush. I was determined to tell everybody – neighbours, friends and casual acquaintances.

When my little sister was born Mummy and Daddy told me she would need help to learn things, more help than I did. Now she can do lots of things and I take her out to play. I think she is lovely.

Where this general advice and counselling have been fol-lowed, surveys show that parents are very satisfied. If parents do not get sensitive help at this critical time, they may fail to seek help later and have difficulty adjusting to their child's handicap (see Chapter 9 on growing up). 'By the time the diagnosis was made Stephen was already a part of the family and we could not consider anything other than keeping him with us.'

The initial surprise and shock do wear off, so what follows in the next chapter covers some of the key areas that may cause fear and doubt in some parents. In addition there are comments and advice from parents who have brought up children with Down's syndrome.

I still feel moments of sadness when I think how much help Timmy needs compared to my other grandchildren, but bit by bit I can see some of the tricks in him that the other children have got up to in the past, and I know I am really glad to have him as part of our family.

5

Help with the baby

Feeding

The decision to breastfeed any baby is a very personal one.
There is no reason why babies with Down's syndrome should
not be successfully breastfed for as long as is necessary;
indeed it may help the mother feel close to her baby in the
beginning.

> I breastfed Katie for nine weeks. I am sure that breastfeed-
> ing creates a wonderful bond between mother and baby,
> and this is particularly helpful in the case of a handicapped
> baby.

This is not to deny that there can be problems with
breastfeeding a baby with Down's syndrome. The poor
muscle tone of the baby can result in the head not being
positioned well in relation to the breast, or the lips may make
an inefficient seal around the nipple. Furthermore, if the
muscle coordination is not as good as it ought to be the action
of swallowing can sometimes be faulty. Certainly, babies with
Down's syndrome often seem to have had enough after only a
short time – obviously less than they need – and although they
often wake and cry for feeds they may just as easily slip back
off to sleep without having taken enough.

When beginning to feed it is therefore important for the
baby to be held fairly upright, and in particular to have the
head supported. It should be checked that the tongue is not
sticking to the roof of the mouth; for a baby to suckle
successfully and get adequate milk, the nipple (or teat, if
bottle feeding) must be on the tongue, not under it. Swallowing can be assisted by supporting the baby's lower jaw with
the fingers and moving it in a rhythmical manner; this also has

the advantage of improving the lip seal.

It is best not to hurry the feed. Babies with Down's syndrome often feed very slowly indeed. As Harriet's mum said, 'Harriet suckled weakly at first, so I kept her alert and awake by tickling her cheeks, chin and feet.'

The baby may also fall asleep at intervals during the feed. It is worthwhile unwrapping the baby, withdrawing the breast or bottle, and changing the nappy before and during the feed.

I managed to breastfeed for four days, but Timothy was a very lazy feeder and it was becoming obvious that he might lose weight. I decided that I would be much happier bottle feeding him as then I could see how much he was getting. Although this was rather difficult Timothy began to gain weight.

Temperature control

In babies with Down's syndrome in particular the body's heat-regulating mechanism does not always work during the early weeks of life, which may in turn contribute to an increased susceptibility to colds and bronchial infections. It is therefore important to ensure that the baby is warm enough, but not too warm.

The bedroom should not feel too cold at night-time, and it should be draught-free. An all-in-one sleeping suit or sleeping bag is useful, as cot blankets and covers can often get kicked off. It is worth remembering that two thin layers of clothing are better than one thick one, and one of the layers can be removed if the baby gets too hot. In cold weather a hat should be worn, even indoors if the house is cold; the head is one of the greatest sources of heat loss.

Skin care

The skin of a baby with Down's syndrome can tend to be very dry. Massaging the skin all over with a little baby oil will help, and will have the advantage of stimulating the baby as well. Baby oil can also be put in the bathwater.

Alternatively a little moisturising cream, e.g. Creme E45, or unperfumed cold cream can be rubbed into the skin every day. This will prevent drying and cracking. Allergic reactions to the creams are rare.

Tongue control

Because of the poor muscle coordination the baby may need special attention to help control the tongue. Playing games such as pulling faces and making noises will all help the child exercise the face and tongue muscles, and will also help with early sounds and, later, with speech. For example, a game could be made of pushing in the tongue over and over again.

As a blocked nose encourages an open mouth and a protruding tongue, an effort should be made to keep it clear.

Developing movement

From the very first weeks after birth the baby should receive lots of encouragement to move. This can be achieved by all sorts of means. For example:

- By bringing the baby into contact with a wide variety of contrasting surfaces – hard and soft, rough/prickly and smooth.
- By handling the baby a lot – with lots of cuddles, tickles hugs and massage.
- By playing with the fingers and toes.

A fuller list of more detailed activities is given on pages 42–3 of this chapter.

Hand/eye coordination

As with any other baby, hand/eye coordination can be developed by providing the baby with Down's syndrome with things to see, touch, feel and listen to, whether in the pram, baby-chair, cot or on the floor. For example, brightly coloured mobiles and musical toys provide good visual interest.

Before our son was born I heard a programme on the radio in which a mother described the achievements of her little girl with Down's syndrome. Our determination to teach our son everything that an ordinary child does naturally has given us endless rewards – the whole family has gained from helping our slow learner.

Damola, our grandson, is the light of our lives. It was a shock to us all when he was born and we were told he had Down's syndrome, but he is now a bright adventurous child going through the 'terrible twos' stage. We are proud of how our daughter and her husband have managed.

Activities

The stimulation of babies from an early stage is an enjoyable introduction to the process of learning. Some suggestions are as follows:

- Blowing on all parts of the baby's body. Tickling, rubbing, patting and gently prodding the baby. Rolling the baby around.
- Lying the baby down naked on a coarse woollen blanket or on crackly paper so that the nerves of the body receive the feel of something different. This can be particularly valuable as an incentive to movement, especially as the sound of the noisy paper is a reward in itself.
- Putting the baby close to the bottom of the cot to encourage pushing against it.
- Placing the baby face down and holding some bright noisy object in front of the eyes and above the head. This will encourage lifting the head to exercise the neck muscles.
- Whistling and singing, using odd sounds that suddenly lapse into a peaceful silence. Any sounds that produce stretches or arching of the back, wriggles or happy twisting.
- Positioning little bells in the cot, not only near the baby's hands but also near (or even on) the feet; this will encourage the baby to kick out more frequently and purposefully. If the bells are placed in the side of the cot the baby may even learn to use alternate limbs.
- Carrying the baby in a sling. In this way the baby is rocked, lowered, lifted and turned in the course of mother's

activity. It will also stimulate the sense of balance and reinforce the feeling of being loved and being part of everything.

- Teasing the baby into making turning, stretching and bending movements by holding some desired object a slight distance away. By making an effort to reach it the baby will learn that effort has its rewards.

- If the baby seems to be making no attempt to crawl, putting a large rolled-up towel in the bath may help. This comfortable bulge will support the chest and abdomen while leaving the limbs free to dangle in the supporting water. Splashing in this position is very close to the movements of crawling.

- It is enjoyable to get down to the same level as the baby to play. By pushing the soles of their feet against the baby's, parents can encourage more active leg movement. The baby can be pulled to standing from this position, or the parent's legs can be used as a ramp to climb.

- Making the baby itch with curiosity by doing something secretive nearby, or clattering about unseen, can make the baby want to overcome the physical stumbling block and get up and find out what is going on.

One parent's view

For me the beginnings of bringing up a slow learner (I prefer this label as it is more hope inspiring than the word handicapped) were not easy. Although the books on baby play were helpful, I still had to feel my way through, especially as my daughter was my first child.

I would let her be close to me a lot; for example, I carried her in a sling, or I wheeled her around the house in a small cot. I propped her up in a slanting chair placed near me on top of the sink or table (ideal for the two of us to look, listen, touch and babble).

I would not let her doze too much, and would not accept this tendency on her part simply as part of 'the condition'. I found that if I made something stand out for her, if I selected for her what she might not have been able to select herself from an overwhelming setting, she showed little sign of tiredness and switching off. Her eyes became alert, her body more tense and her little head less likely to sink loosely into the back of her neck. However, I still respected her need for some switching-off time, as indicated by her remote gaze.

Apart from general babycare, I tried to change the routines. For example I changed her in different places; a bath could be taken in the sink, or with Dad, or in the swimming pool; physical play could occur on a puffy eiderdown or a rough mat.

Parents should not feel compelled to spend a set amount of time in play each day; running a household, particularly if there are other children, is a time-consuming business. Research has shown that as long as the relationship between parents and child is a loving one, then the quality of play and interaction will be good. The quality is probably far more important than the quantity.

Safe, bright and interesting modern toys offer great scope for good quality play. They are designed to delight, provoke and provide enjoyment. If cradle toys are fixed where the feet and knees can kick them, or where the elbows push out, movement is encouraged. It is helpful to use cradle toys made of materials other than plastic, and covered with different textures. Different colours can be used, from pinks and blues to glittering golds and silvers. Wooden toys with clippety-clop sounds, or clicks and clanging cymbals, instead of the usual bell and beady sounds, add variety to experience. Children can be surprised by hanging up a fat balloon, tiny beads, a closed plastic water bag for squeezing, a piece of chocolate, or a mirror. An idea of object permanence can grow out of covering things suddenly and then letting them reappear.

In short, as parents we decided to be on her side, and not make behaviour training our first concern. Looking back, this seems like a daring attitude to have taken, but my now ten-year-old daughter shows me that for her this must have been right.

6

Medical aspects of Down's syndrome

When poor health in Down's syndrome arises it is usually due to maldevelopment of particular organs as a result of processes akin to premature aging or disordered immunity. This chapter will look at specific health problems, and will outline what can be done. Particular emphasis will be placed on heart disease, as this is the commonest cause of poor health in young people with Down's syndrome.

General considerations

Although it does not offer a threat to good health, the skin of children with Down's syndrome is often of concern to parents. The skin tends to be drier than in other children, with a particular tendency to seborrhoeic dermatitis (a dry flakiness or crusting) of the scalp. In cold windy weather the face may become very sore and chapped. The best remedy is the prudent use of a barrier cream, and the addition of oilatum emollient to the bathwater.

Dryness of the skin in some areas of the body can be very marked, with the formation of hyperkeratotic areas (areas of thickened horny skin). Up to 75 per cent of individuals with Down's syndrome will show these, the commoner sites being on the back of the upper arm, including the elbow.

About half the people with Down's syndrome have reddened pimply eruptions, particularly on the trunk, upper thigh and buttock. These areas are actually a dense collection of collagen around normal hair follicles, often with some surrounding inflammation. They can become infected, leading to painful boil and abscess formation, though this is avoidable with appropriate washing and hygiene.

Young people with Down's syndrome also have an increased tendency to alopoecia areata and totalis (patchy bald areas which may come and go, and in some cases total baldness). Vitiligo (areas of reduced skin pigmentation) is also seen more frequently than expected. There are known associations between these disorders and circulating autoantibodies (chemicals produced by the immune system that attack tissues in the body rather than combating infection), although the exact mechanism is unknown. As will be seen in the section on thyroid disorders, it is of interest that people with Down's syndrome have an increase in thyroid autoantibody production too.

Like many children with a disorder of the central nervous system (the brain and spinal cord), there is often relatively poor control of skin blood supply. This often leads to mottling of the skin, in a pattern that corresponds with the pattern of blood vessels. This is particularly evident in the neonatal period, and is known as cutis marmorata. At any age this may lead to the extremities, and in particular the feet and hands, appearing very cold. This rarely seems to give the children themselves any particular concern, but it seems appropriate to use thicker socks on these occasions and make a particular effort to keep gloves on (not always an easy task).

Tears are produced by the lachrymal gland which lies at the inner end of each pair of eyelids. If the tears do not spill over the lower lid on to the cheek, they normally pass down a tunnel, known as the naso-lachrymal duct, to the nose; this is why the nose often needs blowing after crying. Imperfect canalisation of the naso-lachrymal duct is common in Down's syndrome. This leads tears to run down the face rather than into the nose, and may be particularly noticeable in cold and windy weather. The eye may become dry, and infection may lead to a crusting of green-coloured matter around the eyes. Wiping the eyes with saline is the best solution, but if the whites of the eyes become inflamed (conjunctivitis) a course of antibiotic drops may be needed. In the long term, probing of the duct under a short anaesthetic usually relieves the problem.

As in most toddler children, those with Down's syndrome often have a continually runny nose as they pass from one 'cold' (upper respiratory-tract infection) to the next, particularly in winter months. At times the nasal discharge is clear, and at others green or yellow (mucopurulent). Antibiotics should probably be reserved for definite evidence of middle-ear infection (otitis media), lower respiratory tract infection (bronchitis or pneumonia) or when nasal discharge persists for a week. There is generally only a need to take children to the doctor for advice on this when they are clearly ill in themselves, with a persistent high temperature, when they are listless and cannot be bothered to do anything, or if they are tending to pull at one ear. Irritant coughs at night due to catarrh can be eased by the use of sympathomimetic agents which dry up secretions, such as pseudoephedrine.

An irregular dentition is quite common in Down's syndrome, with missing teeth or abnormalities in tooth shape and position. This is another example of poorly canalised developmental pathways (see Chapter 2), leading to an increased variation of normal. Although the incidence of dental caries is lower than in the general population, periodontal (gum) disease is more prevalent. This may be another effect of relatively poor immunity, and makes it particularly important for young children with Down's syndrome to learn about dental hygiene and good teeth cleaning in particular.

The neurology of Down's syndrome – motor abilities

Hypotonia (poor muscle tone) is one of the cardinal features of Down's syndrome. A relative deficiency of excitatory neurotransmitters such as 5-hydroxytryptamine (serotonin), underdevelopment of the cerebellum (one of the motor control centres in the brain), and a generally poor level of dendritic development (see Chapter 2) all play a part. The result is that the neural apparatus in muscles (the muscle spindles and their connections with the spinal cord and brain) is 'set' at too low a level, and muscle tone, particularly in the axis (head and trunk) is poor. Limb tone may be relatively normal, and power at any age is good. The hypotonia generally resolves with age, but there are few adults with Down's syndrome who are not a little hypotonic.

Normal motor development in the first year of life establishes the upright posture. This allows children mobility with their mouth, hands, eyes and ears, free to explore the exciting world and build on their learning experience. Primitive reflexes are imprinted on the central nervous system, from the spinal cord through to brain stem level, facilitating the next developmental step. For example, the asymmetrical tonic neck reflex ensures that every time a baby turns its head the facial hand will be extended before the eyes as a cupid-like posture is adopted. It is quickly learnt that the hand that keeps appearing belongs to the baby, and this knowledge is reinforced and consolidated by visual and tactile information from the mouth.

A number of studies on Down's syndrome have shown that the primitive reflexes in some children persist for longer than expected, while in others they disappear prematurely. Cliff Cunningham's researchers working at the Hester Adrian Research Centre in Manchester showed that intervention before six weeks of age could maintain the presence of the stepping reflex and facilitate early walking. This emphasises that the reciprocal pattern of walking is actually imprinted at a spinal cord level. Interestingly, those children with enhanced cognitive skills (growing intelligence) seemed to fare worst on motor skills. This implies that the two areas of learning are separate, and that there may be a limit to progress in more than one area.

Conflicting results have been reported in relation to the persistence of primitive reflexes, and the relationship motor development has to general development. This serves to emphasise that there are as many differences between people with Down's syndrome as there are in the population as a whole, and that those differences should receive as much emphasis as the similarities.

Physio- and occupational therapists can be very helpful to families in advising them on what to incorporate in play in order to encourage the next developmental stage, particular attention usually being paid to positioning and seating.

The limitation of motor performance in the older child with Down's syndrome comes from an inherent and sometimes severe dyspraxia. This means that, although the muscles, power and strength are present to carry out movement, it is often laboured or clumsy.

People are able to move because they know what a movement feels like. When John McEnroe hits a winning volley he does not have to say to himself that he must pull the racket backwards, transfer his weight on to the back foot, fix the shoulder girdle muscles and so on: he does it because his brain has controlled that movement many times before and is quite capable of building up and computing information from the eyes, ears and sensory equipment in his arms and legs about exactly where his body is in space and exactly what he must do to perform the movement he wishes. In the same way, this is just how we, in a rather less spectacular manner, scratch our noses or put a spoonful of food in our mouths; at first by trial and error, and then with an increasing degree of accuracy.

In Down's syndrome there appears to be a significant problem with this integration of sensory information and the coordination of motor output. The child will be quite aware of what is to be achieved, and will have the equipment to achieve it, but be quite unable to get the movement together. The feedback and integration pathways are qualitatively deficient. In addition, many with Down's syndrome have slow reaction times, a poor ability to dissociate movement (i.e. make one hand do a different thing to the other, as in playing the piano) and difficulty with anticipatory skills and sequencing where the object of the movement is not static (such as hitting a ball). It is probably reaction time, rather than a lack of feeling, which causes children with Down's syndrome to be slow to remove themselves from pain. In these circumstances hot radiators or fingers in a closing door become potentially hazardous and emphasise the need for others to be careful with their advice and with what they do.

These problems of integrating feedback information, and the constant need for adjustment and correction in motor control, are particularly evident in speech. Motor performance in Down's syndrome cannot be regarded as slow normal, but as different (deviating as it does from the usual developmental pathway). This is important for therapists to remember as they devise an individual's intervention programme.

Awkward walking or running is often obvious in Down's syndrome. It is common for the most severely disabled to walk with a fairly stiff-legged gait, and many walk in a valgus (tilting outwards) position at the ankle, with everted (pointed outwards) fore-feet. Where this is severe the question of a spinal cord problem due to atlanto-axial dislocation arises (see later in this chapter). However the presentation of this more serious disorder would be of a deteriorating stiff-legged gait, usually accompanied by bladder or bowel disturbance. In the more severely disabled this may be difficult to define and, where doubt exists, a special X-ray of the spine known as myelography may be the only way of resolving the issue. For the vast majority the observed posture will be no more than the expression of the underlying brain malfunction, and the gait will improve with the sensible use of heel cups and supportive footwear.

Ear abnormality and audiological assessment

Audiological assessment, hearing tests

Any child who has developmental delay, hypotonia and delayed speech and language requires careful assessment to identify the cause of the speech delay, to make sure appropriate services are organised. From time to time children are seen where this has not been carried out 'because the medical diagnosis is obvious'; that is, further assessment is not carried out because it is assumed that the Down's syndrome is the sole cause of the delay. But at least half of children with Down's syndrome will have significant hearing problems.

When sound arrives at the ear, it is funnelled down a canal called the external ear, where it falls on the eardrum (tympanic membrane). The drum vibrates and sends a series of waves of vibration, in time with the sound waves, down a string of three little bones (ossicles) – called the hammer, anvil and stirrup (malleus, incus and stapes). The stirrup is attached to a membrane which forms a window, through which lies the inner ear. The cavity containing the ossicles, between the eardrum and the oval window is known as the middle ear; it is full of air, and is connected to the throat by the Eustachian tube. This is why when ears 'pop' they can be made to feel comfortable again by holding the nose and blowing out hard against a closed throat, forcing air back up the tube into the middle ear. As the stirrup shakes against the oval window, the vibrations are sent on into the inner ear, again in time with the sound that originally formed them.

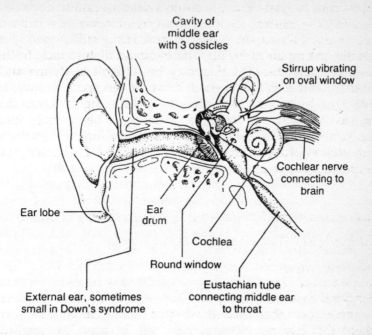

Cavity of
middle ear
with 3 ossicles

Stirrup vibrating
on oval window

Cochlear nerve
connecting to
brain

Ear lobe

Ear
drum

Cochlea

Round window

Eustachian tube
connecting middle ear
to throat

External ear, sometimes
small in Down's syndrome

Diagram of external, middle and internal ear.

The inner ear is a specialised organ called the cochlea; it contains specialised hair-cells that waft in a fluid called lymph. The pattern of vibration formed by the stirrup is picked up by the cochlea hair-cells and transmitted to the brain via the eighth cranial nerve. The temporal lobes of the brain then 'decode' the sound message and make sense of it.

Hearing loss due to a problem in either the external or middle ear is known as conductive deafness: hearing loss due to a problem with the cochlea or its central connections is known as sensorineural or nerve deafness. Conductive loss can often be treated, and can be more often helped with hearing aids; nerve deafness is usually permanent, and is more difficult to help.

The hearing loss in Down's syndrome is sensorineural in 20 per cent of cases, and this incidence increases with age. Up to 50 per cent or so at some stage will have conductive deafness, partly due to anatomical abnormalities in the middle ear and partly due to disordered immunity leading to an increased susceptibility to repeated middle ear infection (see below). One study showed an excessive accumulation of wax in the external ear to be the commonest otological complication of Down's syndrome (31 per cent, versus 14 per cent in other children). Hearing loss in these children averaged 24 decibels (dB). This shows how important it is to be on the lookout for a readily remediable problem.

All children with Down's syndrome should have a formal audiological assessment in infancy and at regular intervals during childhood, the intervals depending on the initial findings. If remedial treatment is not undertaken, a child with hearing loss may develop the secondary problem of poor auditory perception at a cortical level (that is, the brain failing to make sense of what it hears because it has had so little experience of sound, which may in turn affect speech and learning).

One means of assessing how effective any treatment is is to carry out a controlled trial, the results of one form of treatment being compared to those in another group of children (the controls) who have no, or another form of, treatment. It is essential that the results are assessed in an unbiased way, and for this reason the assessor is often not told what treatment has been given (this is a single-blind controlled trial). Sometimes, if the pharmacist has matched the active treatment with a period on a placebo that is identical in appearance but inactive, neither the family nor doctor know what treatment is given (in this case it is a double-blind controlled trial). It is only when these strict scientific rules are followed that we can be absolutely sure that something is effective. Proper assessment is essential, as many treatments are uncomfortable, have side-effects or carry an expense. This subject will be returned to in Chapter 10 on Hopes and Fears.

There have been a number of controlled trials of treatment for conductive deafness due to middle ear effusions (a collection of fluid). It is generally agreed that surgical treatment is indicated where there are bilateral effusions, a persistent subjective hearing loss, a bilateral 25-decibel loss over two or more frequencies, or a bilateral flattening of the tympanogram (measuring how easily the ears 'pop'). A number of studies have shown that adeniodectomy associated

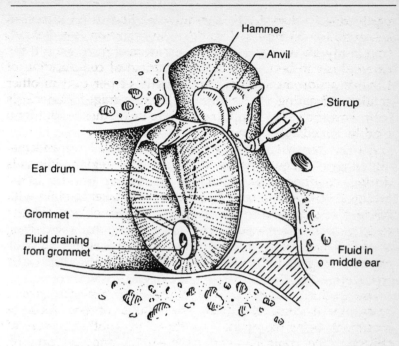

Diagram showing grommets inserted into ear drum draining middle ear.

with myringotomy (making a hole in the drum to let out the fluid) and the insertion of grommets (tiny plastic washers) results in the quickest resolution of both middle ear effusions and infection, and the fastest return of hearing. The majority of the benefit seems to come from the adenoidectomy rather than the insertion of grommets; the long-term effects of grommets are yet to be discerned. One study showed a 40 per cent incidence of a degree of tympanosclerosis (scarring of the drum) after 12 months and a 70 per cent incidence after 21 months. The long-term effects of this on hearing are unknown but, in the majority, tympanosclerosis would seem to be functionally unimportant.

There have been no controlled studies to date on the best treatment of hearing loss in children with Down's syndrome. As the external ear is often so small and narrowed (stenosed), the insertion of grommets may be technically quite difficult. Where the strict selection criteria cited above exist, adenoidectomy is probably still of benefit, but a surgical approach must be complemented by the skilful provision of hearing aids, with appropriate counselling of parents and teachers in their use.

Snoring, a common problem in Down's syndrome, may also be an indication for adenotonsillectomy. Stradling and colleagues from Oxford published a study on 61 snoring children without Down's syndrome. They found that 61 per cent had important degrees of sleep hypoxia (low blood oxygen) and 65 per cent had abnormally disturbed sleep. Many showed daytime sleepiness, hyperactivity, aggression, learning difficulties, restless sleep and odd sleeping positions. Adenotonsillectomy resolved the hypoxia, sleep disturbance and attendant symptoms for the majority. However, careful assessment would be required preoperatively as the presence of abnormal pharyngeal anatomy in Down's syndrome may predispose to postoperative hypernasality (a tendency to speak through the nose).

Eye problems and visual assessment

Eye problems are probably even more common than ear abnormalities. The majority of children with Down's syndrome show a degree of hypermetropia (long-sightedness), though this is often not of a degree that needs correction. Up to 20 per cent may show myopia (short-sightedness) and a smaller percentage astigmatism (an irregular lens, leading to focusing problems in different planes). Screening in infancy should be carried out, with appropriate follow-up. When corrective lenses in the form of spectacles or contact lenses are required, appropriate counselling and support should be offered.

Refractive error may be accompanied by strabismus (squint), and corrective surgery is sometimes required. In up to 5 per cent of cases, congenital cataracts (see Chapter 2) may occur, requiring removal of the diseased lens and the provision of corrective spectacles. Slit lamp examination reveals lens opacities in up to 50 per cent of children with Down's syndrome, this percentage increasing with age. But in the vast majority of cases these are not found in the visual axis and do not interfere with sight.

Specific health problems

Congenital heart and lung disease

Although only one organ, the heart has two distinct halves. The right heart receives blood from the great veins in the body, collects it in the right atrium and then passes it through the tricuspid valve into the right ventricle, a big muscular chamber that pumps blood through the lung (pulmonary) circulation to pick up oxygen. Blood is then returned to the left heart, again to an atrium first and then through the mitral valve into the even larger and more muscular left ventricle, which has the task of pumping the oxygen-laden blood to all the tissues in the body. Normally the right heart and pulmonary circulation is a low pressure system whilst the left heart and the general (systemic) circulation is a high pressure system.

There is normally no connection between the two sides of the heart. If there is an abnormal connection, blood will tend to flow from the high pressure left to the lower pressure right side of the heart. As this blood has already been to the lungs, the child will still normally be pink. This abnormal flow of blood from one side of the heart to the other is known as a shunt. As more blood than usual is now in the lung blood vessels, the pressure in the right side of the heart will go up. It is possible for the pressure to rise so much that it is actually above that in the left side of the heart; this will cause blood to flow in the opposite direction (reverse shunting) and, because it has yet to visit the lungs, it will be low on oxygen, and the child will appear blue (cyanosed).

In the developing foetus the heart starts out as a tube. The tube folds so that the left heart comes to lie slightly above and in front of the right heart. Outgrowths of tissue known as endocardial cushions grow into the cavity of the primitive heart and form the dividing walls (septa) between the two atria and ventricles, a seat for the two valves, an anchor point for the wall that separates the two atria (interatrial septum) and the wall that separates the two ventricles (interventricular septum).

About 40 per cent of children with Down's syndrome have congenital heart disease, and the commonest form is the atrioventricular canal defect. The endocardial cushions are

Diagram of heart development at 4 weeks after conception. Paired tubes on each side have fused to form early right and left atria. Tubes in the midline have joined together and begin to fold to form the bulbo ventricuan tube.

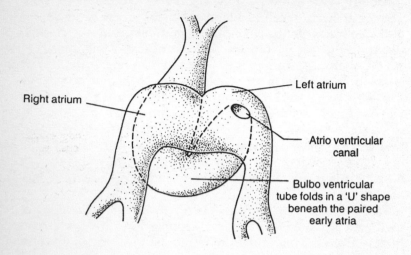

incompletely formed, leading to deficient septa between the atria and ventricles and inefficient mitral and tricuspid valves. Many defects allow initial left-to-right shunting of blood, with a gradual build-up of pulmonary arterial pressure, facilitated on occasions by abnormal pulmonary blood vessels (see below). After some time the resulting pulmonary arterial hypertension (high blood pressure) will reverse the shunt and lead to cyanotic heart disease.

Heart disease may present in the form of a murmur picked up at a routine newborn medical examination; by paroxysmal coughing; or by the presence of breathlessness, particularly at feeding times in the early months or with exercise later. Episodes of pallor and sweating in babies often herald the onset of cardiac failure. About 5 per cent of children with Down's syndrome who have congenital heart disease will have no murmurs initially, and their disease will go unnoticed until the onset of cyanosis, by which time it may be too late for corrective surgery.

For this reason routine echocardiography at a regional centre is recommended for all newborn babies with Down's

Two weeks' later atria and ventricles are formed and the septa grow towards the endocardial cushions which form the seat for the valves.

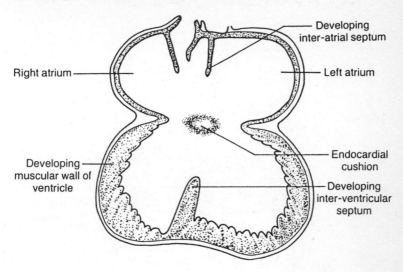

syndrome. This involves checking the heart with a sort of ultra-sound device similar to those used during pregnancy. Where an abnormality is identified, further assessment of the functional consequences will be defined by means of cardiac catheterisation. The information this yields will allow a rational decision on the timing of intervention to be taken. Cardiac catheterisation involves feeding a small tube along a vein or artery to the heart and measuring the pressures in the different chambers. Dye may also be injected so that the anatomy can be defined using X-rays.

Congenital heart disease accounts for 30 to 35 per cent of deaths in Down's syndrome, and the mortality is highest in the first two years of life. Chest infections account for approximately the same number of deaths, but it is conceivable that a congenital cardiac defect may contribute to some of these cases.

The lung consists of millions of tiny air-cells called alveolae, which are very rich in capillaries to help the diffusion of oxygen into the blood. Some children with Down's syndrome are born with hypoplastic (underdeveloped) lungs, with

Complete heart development with separate right and left atria and right and left ventricles.

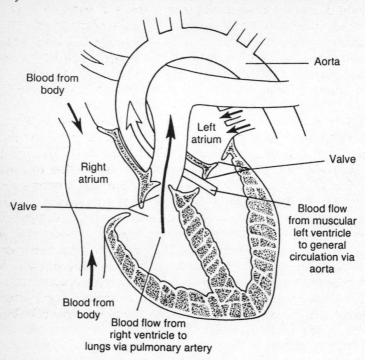

structural changes specific to Down's syndrome. The double capillary network on the alveolar wall, normal in foetal life, persists. The alveolar ducts are increased in size, but the number of alveolae and their surface area is reduced. These abnormalities predispose children with heart disease to pulmonary hypertension, and the increased blood flow due to the large arteriovenous shunt also predisposes to chest infection. An inefficient body defence (immune) system may add to this tendency.

A decision needs to be made, irrespective of the child's ability, on whether to attempt surgical correction. The decision-making process should involve a lot of discussion between the parents and medical team, to share knowledge and weigh up the advantages and disadvantages of the different options available in individual cases. Sometimes temporary solutions can be found such as 'banding' the pulmonary artery; the surgeon applies a band around the vessel, making it far more difficult for the blood to flow to the lungs. It then takes the easier route into the left heart and on to the general circulation, while the lungs are protected from the excessive volumes of blood that lead to secondary pulmonary hypertension. The more definitive corrective surgery can then be carried out at a later date.

A conservative policy, using purely medical as opposed to surgical treatment, guarantees a far higher rate of childhood survival. Affected people are likely to live on to their third or fourth decade, when death inevitably strikes due to cardiac failure or concomitant lung disease. Surgical treatment still carries a high mortality, with early post-operative death rates at 20 to 30 per cent in many centres. Even after surgery there may be a residual anomaly, yet surgery remains the only chance to avoid the crippling pulmonary vascular disease.

The mainstay of medical treatment remains digoxin and diuretics for cardiac failure, beta-blockade for cyanotic attacks due to pulmonary artery spasm, and antibiotic prophylaxis to cover dental procedures so that bacterial endocarditis (infection of the heart) might be avoided.

Thyroid disorders and growth

The thyroid gland is to be found just beneath the Adam's apple (actually called the thyroid cartilage). It is an endocrine gland and, as such, produces a number of thyroid hormones, principally thyroxine (T4) and tri-iodothyronine (T3), both of which govern the rate of body metabolism. Overactivity of the gland leads to overactive cells, the increased consumption of energy and loss of weight as reserves are 'burnt-up'. Conversely, an underactive gland will lead all the biochemical reactions and processes in the body to slow down; the result will be less call on energy sources, and weight gain. Thyroid hormones are also essential for normal growth, and deficiency will lead to short stature. Brain nerve cells are reliant on thyroid hormones for normal activity, so mental deficiency can result from underactivity of the gland.

Neonatal thyroid abnormalities are very rare in Down's

syndrome. In one study 12 out of 1,130 patients had thyroid dysfunction, but in four of these it was transient; the remainder had primary hypothyroidism, which should be identified by neonatal screening programmes now being adopted by many regional health authorities. Persistent hypotonia (head, trunk and limbs), good weight gain despite very poor feeding, prolonged jaundice, dry skin, sparse hair and a hoarse cry are all signs of this disorder. Some of these symptoms overlap with the characteristics of Down's syndrome, but when doubt exists blood should be taken for thyroid function tests.

The main advent of thyroid disfunction is in the teenage years. In one study from Glasgow four out of 116 children were found to have thyroid disease; three were hypothyroid and one was hyperthyroid. About a third of them were found to have thyroid autoantibodies, and this has been reported in other studies. The matter needs further evaluation, but it would seem sensible to screen children with Down's syndrome with thyroid function tests, and for the presence of thyroid autoantibodies at about the age of ten, and then at intervals thereafter depending on the results of those investigations. It is not yet known what percentage of children with thyroid autoantibodies proceed and develop functional thyroid disorders, and in what percentage it is merely a transient phenomenon.

Unnoticed hypothyroidism has been shown to have an adverse effect on intellectual performance. Pueschel, from Rhode Island Hospital, USA, has written extensively on Down's syndrome. He studied 151 young people with Down's syndrome and showed there was an increasing tendency with age for thyroid stimulating hormone (TSH) levels to rise as thyroxine (T4) levels fell. He compared the IQ of those with abnormal TSH and T4 to those with increased TSH alone, and to those with normal thyroid function tests. The results were 41.77, 53.8 and 55.3 respectively. Although Koch in 1965, in a double-blind study, found no benefit from the random administration of thyroxine, these data from Pueschel make a strong case for regular screening and appropriate treatment.

Growth retardation is a feature of Down's syndrome, and data exist on growth in 730 children, based on 4,650 observations up to the age of 18 years to allow assessment of growth in children with the syndrome. Another endocrine gland, the pituitary, which lies just below and has close connections with the fore-brain, is responsible for the production of a number of growth factors. These include human growth hormone and the somatomedins. They, like insulin, encourage cells to take up energy sources like glucose from the blood and have an anabolic (building-up) effect on body metabolism.

Children with Down's syndrome show a deficiency in serum insulin-like growth factor (IGF-1). This growth-hormone-dependent somatomedin fails to rise during childhood, and remains at a low concentration throughout life. The serum concentration of insulin-like growth factor 2 (IGF-2) in patients with Down's syndrome is normal, and somatomedin and insulin receptors are also normal. A number of children have been described who have shown abnormalities of growth over and above that expected in a population of children with Down's syndrome. These children have responded to treatment with human growth hormone. The decision to treat, however, is not straightforward; growth hormone treatment increases the risk of leukaemia (see below), and the reason for treatment should always be well defined and understood from the child's point of view. There is no evidence that growth hormone increases learning ability.

Gonadotrophins (the sex hormones) will be reviewed in Chapter 9. From that discussion, and from data on thyroid and growth hormone function, it can be deduced that the biological activity of these hormones may be reduced. Although testicular failure in some males is primary, and auto-immune thyroiditis is an important cause of hypothyroidism, other factors are probably important. The research is yet to be done, but it is likely that target-organ failure plays a role in endocrine hypofunction. In target-organ failure there is adequate hormonal production but the 'target tissues' on which the hormones usually act fail to respond. The common factor may well be a disorder of membrane metabolism.

Skeletal abnormalities

Skull and middle-ear shape, and the possible effect on hearing, have already been considered. Absence of the 12th rib, incomplete fusion of the lower spinal vertebral arches, and fusion of the second and third toes are well described associations with Down's syndrome.

In recent years the top two bones in the spinal column, the atlas and the axis, have received a lot of attention. The spinal column is really a stack of bones, called vertebrae, which stand on top of each other. There is a hole down the middle of each, through which passes the spinal cord – a long cylinder containing millions of nerve cells transmitting messages for motor activity from the brain to muscles in the arms, legs and trunk, and gathering sensory information on pain, temperature, joint position and so on and sending it back up to the brain. The atlas and the axis vertebrae, at the top of the spinal column, are very different in shape. The atlas supports the base of the skull above it, and its saucer shape allows nodding movement of the skull. The atlas has a large hole in its centre through which part of the axis, the odontoid peg, protrudes; this allows pivoting side-to-side movement. All these vertebrae are joined by ligaments and muscles, but in Down's syndrome the ligaments tend to be lax and the muscle tone tends to be poor. This allows undue movement between the atlas and axis, and raises the danger of the odontoid peg squashing the spinal cord which lies just behind it.

This movement of the atlas on the axis is referred to as atlanto-axial dislocation, or subluxation. The Department of Health has issued guidance on children with Down's syndrome likely to undertake physical activity which might put them at increased risk of subluxation. This includes the hyperextension of the neck which occurs during the induction of anaesthesia, when a tube is passed into the wind-pipe.

Hospital-based studies indicate that there is undue movement of the odontoid peg relative to the atlas (4.5 mm or more) in up to 20 per cent of people with Down's syndrome, with a certain improvement as children get older. Despite the frequency of the phenomenon, only 15 cases of spinal cord damage had been described in the 22-year-period up to 1987. In the author's experience X-rays of the neck are unreliable in showing instability, and given the very small risk involved it is probably not worth screening children with Down's syndrome in this way. Common sense should apply, and anaesthetists be appraised of the risks of anaesthesia and parents appraised of the risks their children run when pursuing more active sports such as trampolining and high-diving.

This is now the basis of current Department of Health guidance. It is no longer a requirement to screen for atlanto-axial instability and many young people with Down's syndrome who were previously excluded from sporting events can now enjoy the benefit of participation.

Gastrointestinal abnormalities

Constipation is a common symptom in Down's syndrome. Poor muscle tone, mobility and fluid intake probably all contribute, especially in young babies. The symptom tends to improve, as all these things improve, with age. Attention should be paid to an adequate amount of fluid intake and roughage in the diet.

Babies may be helped to open their bowels by gently inserting a cotton-bud coated with petroleum jelly a short distance into the anus (back passage). For older children, if the bowels have not opened for, say, three days, a glycerine suppository usually helps. If the difficulty persists the family doctor may wish to prescribe medication which keeps the stools soft, or laxatives.

Developmental abnormalities of the intestines are rare in Down's syndrome, but are most likely to present in the newborn period. Duodenal atresia is the commonest. The duodenum is the first part of the folded tube-like structure known as the intestine. The intestines begin at the stomach and end at the anus; their job is to break down and absorb food, a process called digestion. Atresia means the tube has failed to canalise properly so that the stomach is passing its contents on into a blind ending cul-de-sac.

Duodenal atresia presents with vomiting (as there is a build-up of milk) and absolute constipation (as no food can pass the blockage). Unlike other forms of intestinal obstruction there is no abdominal distension as the blockage is at the beginning of the bowel which cannot therefore become distended with gas. There may or may not be bilious vomiting, depending on whether the atresia has arisen before or after the bile duct enters the duodenum. There is often a history of polyhydramnois (more fluid than usual around the

growing baby in the amniotic sac) because the normal flow of
amniotic fluid through the baby's intestines has been disrupted. A plain abdominal X-ray reveals the characteristic 'double
bubble' of gas in the stomach and first part of the duodenum.
After initial resuscitation, corrective surgery can be carried
out.

Malabsorption (poor absorption of nutrients from the
intestine) is now recognised as a problem in some people with
Down's syndrome. Recently there have been reports of an
increased incidence of coeliac disease. This is an immune-
mediated disorder in which an allergy is developed to the
gliadin fraction of gluten in wheatgerm. The intestinal mucosa
becomes inflamed and then atrophies (undergoes a significant
degree of shrinkage). The absorptive surface is then reduced,
and malabsorption results. Treatment is with a gluten-free
diet that leads to recovery of the mucosal surface of the bowel.

Specific malabsorption of vitamin B12 has also been
reported in a three-year-old girl with Down's syndrome. She
presented with loss of weight, diarrhoea, day-time wetting,
cold peripheries, lethargy, loss of appetite and a rash. A
peripheral blood count showed the large red cells (macrocytosis) typical of B12 deficiency, and a Schilling test confirmed
this was due to malabsorption. Unlike other reported cases
she did not have protein in her urine. She made a good
recovery with B12 injections. There have been no other
reported cases so far, and it may never be repeated, but it does
serve to emphasise the importance of not attributing all
symptomatology to the syndrome itself.

Disordered immunity/leukaemia

People with Down's syndrome have poorly functioning
immune systems; they have relatively poor responses to
infections and tend to mount inappropriate attacks on their
own bodies. This is a very active area of research, and this
section will highlight some of the important developments.

One of the most important components of human immunity
are the T-cell lymphocytes; so-called because they are produced in the thymus gland, which is found in the upper part
of the chest. It is their job to recognise invading substances as
'not-self', in which case they multiply rapidly to form clones

of cells that neutralise the invader.

It is suggested that there is an intrinsic T-cell immune defect in Down's syndrome which is responsible for the increased susceptibility to malignancy, infection and auto-immune disorders (see above under thyroid function). In the laboratory T cells can be made to multiply in a non-specific way with the use of a substance called phytohaemagglutinin (PHA). In Down's syndrome this appears to be normal for the first 10 years of life, and then declines. More specific reactions can be studied with the use of monoclonal antibodies (very specific invading proteins) such as anti-CD3. The response of lymphocytes in Down's syndrome in this situation is significantly reduced at any age. Studies have shown that this is not due to the T-cells being unable to latch on to (bind to) the foreign protein, nor to defective interaction with monocytes which 'mop-up the debris'. Instead overexpanded populations of specialised T-cells which limit and confine the immune response have been found. These are called suppressor and natural killer cells. The problem may then be due to excess numbers (another gene dose effect) of inhibitory immunoregulatory cells.

One can speculate that the inefficient response may also be due to the abnormalities of membrane function. The T lymphocytes of younger people with Down's syndrome have significantly elevated levels of cyclic guanine monophosphate, a substance which acts as a substrate for an enzyme called guanylate cyclase, which in turn is very important for normal membrane and cell wall function. In this respect they resemble cells of older normal people and the immunodeficient state that accompanies aging.

Lymphocyte functional antigen-1 (LFA-1) assists the binding of immune lymphocytes to antigens. A large part of this substance is coded for at 21q22. Again, because of the gene-dosage effect, LFA-1 is seen in increased levels on Down's syndrome cells. This leads the lymphocytes to show increased adhesiveness, with resulting non-specific binding. The immune response therefore lacks a degree of specificity, and becomes inefficient.

The cell surface receptor for an important substance called interferon, produced against viruses, is coded for on chromosome 21. This leads the sensitivity to the anti-viral effects of interferon to be several-fold greater in Down's syndrome, even though interferon production is the same. It is possible that people with Down's syndrome are more susceptible to viral infection because this sensitivity of the interferon receptors to the immunosuppressive effects of interferon leads to a premature shutdown of the response.

This impairment of cell-mediated immune reactions probably leads to inefficient immunosurveillance (the T-cells search and destroy any substance that is foreign, abnormal or 'not-self'). An increased susceptibility to infection tends not to be of great clinical importance after infancy, although increased numbers of skin and middle-ear infections are reported. One popular misconception is that people with Down's syndrome are at risk of contracting hepatitis B (the type contracted from blood products). This is not the case, although hepatitis A (infectious hepatitis) used to be quite prevalent in institutions, which is probably how the misunderstanding arose.

Although increased risk of infection is not of great practical importance the 1 per cent reported incidence of leukaemia is 14-fold higher than in the general population. Robison and colleagues from the US Children's Cancer Study Group reported their findings on 5,406 children with acute lymphoblastic (ALL) and non-lymphoblastic leukaemia (ANLL) in 1984. Two per cent of the patients had Down's syndrome. The children with Down's syndrome showed a lower remission rate (81 per cent versus 94 per cent), a greater induction (beginning of treatment) mortality (14 per cent versus 3 per cent), and a significantly lower five-year survival (50 per cent versus 65 per cent). In the UK the outlook for five-year survival seems even worse (28 per cent versus 59 per cent). The Americans reported that if initial remission was achieved, then there was no significant difference with respect to duration, survival or disease-free interval, between children with Down's syndrome and other children.

Children with Down's syndrome seem to fare worse because of their susceptibility to infection and the vulnerability of their bone-marrows to the drugs used in therapy. They are particularly sensitive to the antifolate agents and methotrexate in particular. In general only 30–50 per cent of the standard dose is tolerated. In spite of this the Great Ormond Street group advocate that, where possible, standard chemotherapeutic regimens should be used to give the best chance of success, but that this requires 'aggressive support'. In other words, to improve the chance of survival, children with Down's syndrome often have to be made really quite ill in the course of their therapy.

Epilepsy

Epilepsy is more common in Down's syndrome than in the general population, but nevertheless remains relatively rare, affecting between 1 and 5 per cent. Those children who develop epilepsy tend to be the more severely intellectually impaired, but there are notable exceptions to this rule. As in all other children with epilepsy, the character of the seizure type must be defined by means of a detailed history, assessment and EEG (electroencephalographic) recordings. An EEG is performed with the child wearing a sort of 'crown' on the head for 10 to 15 minutes, the electrodes in the crown detecting electrical activity in the brain. The pattern of electrical activity allows the doctor to decide if there is any evidence of epilepsy and, if so, just what form it takes. From this information, advice on outlook and the most appropriate form of therapy can be given.

Some of the drugs used to treat epilepsy, like anti-cancer drugs, interfere with folate metabolism; because of this, long-term effects on the blood count and bone metabolism need to be monitored on an annual basis.

Aging Alzheimer's disease

Alzheimer's disease is the most common form of pre-senile dementia in Britain, affecting 5 per cent of the population over 65 and 20 per cent over the age of 80. It accounts for 50 per cent of those with dementia in the general population. Pathologists can diagnose the condition when they see specific appearances on brain biopsy; these are neuritic plaques and neurofibrillary tangles.

Particular neuronal systems are affected, involving the memory and cognitive systems found in a part of the brain called the hippocampus, and its cortical connections. As this neuronal loss is selective, a problem involving specific neuro transmitters can be ruled out, although a deficiency of cholinergic nerve cells has been demonstrated. The neuritic plaques have a core of protein mixed with aluminium silicates, dystrophic (abnormally grown) neurites and neuro-glia (cells that support nerve-cells in the brain). There is an association between aluminium and Alzheimer's disease, but there is no clear dose-related trend. The difference in bioavail-ability of aluminium from differing sources may be important, as may genetic susceptibility; more clinical and epidemiologi-cal studies are needed. The proteinaceous material in the core seems to be A4 or beta-amyloid, the gene coding for this lying on the long arm of chromosome 21. It seems most likely that a gene dosage effect for this peptide is not causative but rather that the Alzheimer's disease locus lies close to that of A4-amyloid within band 21q21.

The disease is particularly common in Down's syndrome and increasingly so after the age of 40. Some authors have claimed that people with Down's syndrome inevitably develop the disease eventually, but others dispute this. Early manifestations are an insidious loss of memory and intellec-tual function which lead to confusion, disorientation and ultimately to profound mental and physical disability.

The diagnosis is made by excluding other conditions that lead to confusional states and dementia. Computerised tomo-graphic (CT) scanning can be helpful in excluding other causes, although the appearances are very often non-specific and multiple infarct dementia, so common in the elderly, is rare in Down's syndrome because of the rarity of atheroma (see Chapter 2). Magnetic resonance imaging (MRI) gives better resolution of white matter changes in the brain, but the technique is not widely available and the scanning time is considerably longer than for CT scanning. For a confused person with a learning disability this would often require a general anaesthetic. Positron emission tomography (PET) scanning reveals functional changes at a biochemical level, and in one recent study was shown to be more useful than the other two techniques in terms of reflecting the degree of pathology. Study of neurotransmitters in cerebrospinal fluid gives non-specific results and the electroencephalogram (EEG) is unhelpful. Clinical evaluation by a caring and astute physician remains the mainstay of investigation of people with learning difficulties who develop dementia.

Various attempts have been made at replacement therapy, concentrating particularly on the deficient cholinergic system. In addition to using the acetyl-choline precursors choline and lecithin, anticholinesterases and receptor agonists have been used. Anticholinesterases boost the naturally occurring levels of acetyl-choline, while agonists boost its effect. Trials had not shown any important benefits until 1986, when Summers reported significant improvement in some patients with the use of tetra-hydro-aminoacridine (THA). THA is a potent centrally-acting anticholinesterase and stimulant; it increases the need for free choline and in some trials it has been given with lecithin. As with all anticholinergics, it can give unwanted gastrointestinal effects and hypotension. More seriously, in up to a third it can cause hepatotoxicity (liver damage) due to a chronic hepatitis. This is said to be reversible on stopping the drug, but further evaluation of its risks and benefits are needed.

Meanwhile a pragmatic approach to therapy has to be adopted. The major tranquillisers can bring calmness to the very disturbed, but side-effects may be troublesome. More importantly, a close liaison needs to be established between learning difficulty support services who comfort those affected and their families. Research continues into the causes and treatment of this common disorder.

7

Going to school

Young children with Down's syndrome who have been taught and encouraged from their earliest days benefit from attending a local playgroup or nursery school before going on into the full-time educational system. They should also enjoy the activities undertaken by other children of the same age, such as ballet classes, swimming and horseriding. However, it is often the search for an appropriate nursery placement that first brings parents into contact with their local education authority (LEA).

The LEA and statements of special educational need

The 1981 Education Act was an important step towards ensuring a right to integration in mainstream education for children with special needs. The Act also established the duty of education authorities to identify those children for whom it was necessary to make a statement and to assess what help was needed for each child.

The 1993 Education Act built on these foundations and instituted the Special Educational Needs Tribunal, a body independent from the LEAs to which parents may appeal against certain decisions of the LEA. The current law setting out the duties and responsibilities of LEAs, Governors and Schools to pupils with special educational needs is now set out in the Education Act 1996.

An officer of the Local Education Authority (LEA) carries out a formal assessment to assess a child's strengths and weaknesses. They are required to seek advice from a number of professional sources as well as from the parent. A statement of special educational needs is then drawn up identifying the needs of the child and specifying the special educational provision to meet those needs. Provision for nursery nurses or non-teaching assistants is commonly made, to supervise the activity of children with learning difficulties in the classroom and at breaktime, along with the provision of appropriate remedial therapy such as speech therapy. Unless the parent makes suitable arrangements themselves the LEA has a legal duty to arrange that the special educational provision set out in the statement is made for the child.

Unfortunately the duty to educate children with special educational needs in mainstream school is only a qualified duty. As well as being compatible with the child receiving the necessary special educational provision, integration must be compatible with the efficient education of the other children in the school and the efficient use of resources. Local authorities have not had a uniform approach to their duty to educate children in mainstream schools and the limitations on the duty have been relied on in some areas to justify children being accommodated in special schools, when integration in mainstream school would have been a valid option.

Parents may ask for an assessment of their child at any stage. Before their child is 2 years old, if it is necessary for their special educational provision to be decided by the LEA, the LEA may make an assessment with the consent of the parent – and is duty bound to do so at the parents' request. Such assessment and any statement made are not subject to the formal process that the law requires when the child is over 2.

The LEA may learn of a child's special educational needs from their doctor who has a duty to tell the parent and then the education authority of any child under 5 who has (or probably has) special educational needs.

After the age of 2 the LEA has a duty to identify those children with special needs whose special educational provision they need to decide. The LEA must notify parents if they propose to assess their child and give parents 29 days in which to comment. If parents request an assessment for a child over 2 the LEA must comply if it is necessary to make an assessment and there has not been one in the past six months. If the LEA refuses to assess following such a request the parent may appeal to the Special Educational Tribunal.

Parents must receive notice of any examination of their

child for the purpose of the assessment and have a right to be present. Parents who refuse to take their child for an assessment or examination without a reasonable excuse commit an offence and can be prosecuted and fined.

The assessment must generally be completed within ten weeks of the LEA's decision to make an assessment. Within a further two weeks the LEA must either notify the parent of their decision not to make a statement and the parents right to appeal to the Special Educational Tribunal against this decision or send to the parent a copy of the proposed statement.

The proposed statement will be in the same form and with the same contents as the LEA plan to put into the final statement except that Part 4 will be blank instead of naming the school the child is to attend. Parents then have an opportunity to let the LEA know their views on the contents of the statement and express a preference for the maintained or grant maintained school they want for their child. Parents views (known as representations) and the name of their preferred school must be sent to the LEA within 15 days of receiving the statement unless the parents exercise their right to request a meeting with an officer to discuss the statement. If a meeting is called and parents are still unhappy they can request a further meeting to discuss any of the professional advice with an appropriate person. Where parents request a meeting the 15 days within which to make representations or express a preference for a school, runs from the date of the meeting or the further meeting if one is requested. The final statement should be made within eight weeks of sending the proposed statement. Parents can appeal to the Special Educational Needs Tribunal against the contents of the final statement including the school named. All appeals to the Special Educational Needs Tribunal must be made within two months from the LEA notifying the parents of their right to appeal.

After statements are made they must be reviewed within 12 months. Different rules apply to the first annual review following the child's fourteenth birthday, which begins to plan for the child's adult life by drawing up a transition plan.

The recent educational climate has caused some concern to parents of children with special educational needs. The baseline of the national curriculum will not be obtainable by all children with Down's syndrome. Discussions are continuing with the SCAA (Schools Curriculum and Assessment Authority) about a suitable curriculum for those who are severely learning impaired.

There is anxiety that mainstream schools will be less inclined to accommodate children with special educational needs because of their likely effect on school league tables. Special educational provision for children with Down's syndrome can be expensive and where schools are holding their own budget they can see such children as a charge on their resources, particularly where the statement is not sufficiently specific to commit the LEA to any expenditure.

A school's attitude to special education can be considerably influenced by the governing body. Governors have a duty to do their best to secure special educational provision for children with learning difficulties in their schools. With this in mind it is clearly of advantage to parents of children with Down's syndrome to get themselves elected to the governing bodies of schools.

Many officers of LEAs, educational authorities and head-teachers are very sympathetic and supportive to the ideal of integration.

When parents are first thinking about finding a playschool or school for their children, they are well advised to visit as many establishments as possible in the area. The final choice is often a difficult one, and in the end is based on a mixture of factors including the previous experience a school has of children with special needs, perceived attitude of the staff and geographical location. At times parents will feel hurt when they come up against headteachers who seem to lack understanding, but persistence coupled with the philosophy behind the Education Act and the goodwill of most professionals will usually secure success in the end.

SUMMARY OF PROCEDURES

Children under 2
- Parent can ask for assessment.
- District Health Authority must tell parent, then Educational Authority, that child may have special educational needs.

- Education Authority may (with consent of parent) and must (at request of parent) make an assessment which can be of any kind, and may result in a Statement of Special Educational Needs.

Children between 2 and 19
- Authorities have a duty to identify children whose special educational needs make it necessary for the authority to decide on special educational provision.
- Parents can request assessment and authorities cannot unreasonably refuse.
- Parents can appeal against refusal to assess.

Assessment
- Notice to parents – 29 days to comment.
- If authority decides not to assess, must notify parent.
- Parents must receive notices of any examinations; have a right to be present and to submit information.
- Parents who fail to see that their children turn up for examinations without reasonable excuse may be guilty of offence and fined.

After assessment
- Authority may decide not to make statement, may issue a Note in Lieu of a Statement instead.
- Must inform parents of right of appeal to SEN Tribunal.
- If authority decides to make statement, must serve copy of proposed statement on parents and enable parents to state a preference for a school.
- Parents have 15 days in which to express a preference and make representations or ask for meeting with officer, and a further 15 days to ask for other meetings with professionals to discuss professional advice provided to authority (which must be given to parents as part of statement).
- Authority, after considering parents' views, can make statement in the same or changed form (but must include name of school in statement) or decide not to make it; must inform parents.
- If statement is made, must be sent to parents with notice of right to appeal in writing to SEN Tribunal, which can confirm statement, or ask LEA to reconsider it.

After Statement is made
- Statements must be reviewed within every 12 months.
- Young people aged 14+ must have a Transition Plan drawn

up after each Annual Review.

- Parents can appeal if the Statement is amended or if there is a decision to cease to maintain the statement, or a refusal to name a different school.
- The LEA must see that special educational provision set out in statement is made.

Liaison

One of the keys to a child's success and happiness is that parents, therapists, carers and staff in the school or in clinics liaise with each other so that aims and achievements can be coordinated as much as possible. In this respect parents have a key role, but they often appreciate the support and advocacy of one of the pre-school support team members in establishing links with education, health or social services.

If parents have been encouraging their child since birth through natural play guided by therapists, they will want to continue this process by reinforcing the activities that are taught at playschool, and later at primary school. Children with Down's syndrome will often not be able to report clearly what they experience at school and this makes close liaison essential, especially if remedial therapists are involved; regular discussions on a child's developments and achievements at home and at school are often enlightening for parents and staff alike. Communication logs, daily diaries or home/school books can be helpful in this respect, in which both parents and teachers may keep a record of significant events.

Some parents may feel apprehensive about contacting 'professionals' in this way, or even about asking teachers and nursery school staff to take their child in the first place. Some may expect a more structured teaching programme than is actually provided. In all these cases it is important for contact to be made with the relevant people. Invariably staff will be more than willing to meet the needs of each child and family.

On a more practical level, if the child has a heart defect it is important that everyone is made aware of this and of the limitations it may place on activity. A school nurse should be involved, and contact between the school, hospital and community paediatricians and the family doctor are particularly helpful. In general, though, activity should be limited as little as possible so as to increase independent confidence and a sense of belonging.

If school staff have only a broad knowledge of Down's syndrome, they may feel that the list of physical needs is rather daunting. But they ought to realise that not all children with Down's syndrome have all the problems at once, if at all. Many children will already have learned to cope with any problems in their own way by the time they get to school age. Staff should be prepared to learn from the child, with obvious benefit. In the classroom the Down's syndrome becomes irrelevant. Each child's individual strengths and weaknesses need assessment.

Finally it should be remembered that a move from the relative shelter of home to nursery school or playschool, or from nursery school to infant school and then to primary school, can be a big step for any child. Parents should if possible visit the school on a number of occasions with the child, so as to give them a chance to look around and help them feel comfortable with their new environment.

Preparation

While it is obviously helpful for the staff at playschool or school if a child can recognise their own peg, cope with dressing, undressing, toileting and so on, these are not skills that are necessary to start with. Overemphasis on this sort of issue can lead to overanxiety in children and their parents. Children learn quickly from other children; children with Down's syndrome often find copying very easy and are likely to pick up what is required of them quite quickly. However, a few practical hints which may be of use are:

- Garments should be labelled with the child's name, to help easy identification in busy cloakrooms.
- Clothes can be trendy but not 'best', as they are liable to get paint splashed on them, or pulled during boisterous play.
- Clothes that are easy to remove for going to the toilet are advisable – avoid dungarees with complicated fastenings.
- Ski-pants or track-suit bottoms allow a child to crawl around on cold floors without getting scuffed knees and cold legs.

CLOSS Visit Notes   Mon 5th Nov

During the course of this visit I played 2 group games with Michael as follows;

Find it

Perception Lotto. - Each child has a picture & then has to find smaller picture cards within their picture. Michael enjoyed this and tried very hard to find the pictures, (he had a house). He found the larger items e.g. bicycle easy and the smaller pictures more difficult e.g. goldfish bowl. This was no different to the problems experienced by all the children I played this with.

Coloured Cube Designs

This consisted of cube designs and wooden cubes to copy the designs with. Once again, like the other children Michael found it relatively easy to place the cubes in the correct places on the cards but extremely difficult to copy the design below the card.

When I left Michael was absorbed in completing quite a complicated inset puzzle.

I will run a Makaton session next Mon lunchtime.

J. Greic.

Sample of note written by one of the teachers in a complex learning difficulties support service for parents at home.

- Tops should have sleeves that can be pushed up the arms easily, with no cuff bottoms. This allows paint and water play without the child getting soaked.
- Long hair should be tied back, partly to keep it out of the way, but also to discourage other children from playing with their new friend like a doll.

In the classroom.

It is important to introduce children to their new nursery staff or teachers. They are bound to be apprehensive about being left to start with. Parents are often allowed to stay a short time in the introductory days, and it can be helpful to leave a familiar object for comfort.

As the child's concept of time is poor it helps if teachers explain that the child's mother and father will be coming back after a certain activity or event, for example 'When lunch is ready', 'After lunch', 'After you have made a picture'. The description should be accurate, and the teacher should ensure that what has been described really is the last activity or event of the school day. Children with Down's syndrome often understand instructions literally and if a parent is supposed to be arriving after a child 'has made a picture', and the day's events are not programmed, the child may do nothing more once the picture is finished and remain rather confused about why it is not time to go home.

Social skills

The ability range in Down's syndrome, although lower and generally slower, is as wide as in any other group of children. It always bears repeating that facial appearance gives no indication of that individual child's ability or potential. It is worth emphasising that much of a child's personality is determined by their home and family background, as much as chromosomal make-up.

A popular misconception is that children with Down's syndrome are always lovable and affectionate. Some are, but only some of the time. All children can be annoying at times, behave badly and be disobedient or easily distracted; children with Down's syndrome are no exception. However, children with Down's syndrome can get into difficulties in their efforts to help or be friendly; for example they may greet people in what may be an inappropriate way by kissing or hugging. This tendency gets better as social rules are learnt through observing the behaviour of other children. Adults should treat a child with Down's syndrome as they would all other members of the class or group. Classmates, too, need to be encouraged to interact normally both in and out of school; there is often a tendency to 'mother', as the child with Down's syndrome is seen to be vulnerable. Children at school age are very sensitive to other children's ability, and naturally feel protective and supportive if they sense a child is less able than they are. If the reaction of others is appropriate, children with Down's syndrome will learn confidence, encouragement and independence.

Behaviour

Staff at playschool or school may have no previous experience of Down's syndrome, but just the same misconceptions that confronted the parents at the time of the child's birth. It is therefore helpful if parents paint a picture of their child for the teachers in the reception class, as misunderstandings are far easier to prevent than to undo.

Many children with Down's syndrome have long memories, particularly for events and people, which leads them to be routine conscious and quite resistant to change. This leads them to be easily upset if explained plans or the usual routine is unexpectedly changed. Whenever possible changes in staffing or activity that can be foreseen should be explained and presented in a positive manner. Children with Down's syndrome are often described as being stubborn. In fact they can often become very engrossed in the simplest of tasks, putting on socks or drawing a picture, and when asked to perform a different activity display temporary frustration. Confrontation is best avoided and if simple explanation does not work then imaginative distraction is called for; an attempt to make them laugh often works.

Stages of development usually last longer in any child with learning difficulties. This means that irritating habits may take more than the expected time to be extinguished. Sometimes children with Down's syndrome go through a stage when they repeat what is said to them in an effort to please rather than because what they are saying is true. They may answer 'Yes' when they actually mean 'No', with the correct answer probably following on after a brief pause.

A strong sense of humour and a mischievous streak are often features of children with Down's syndrome. This love of mischief, if combined with boredom, can lead to inconvenient attention-seeking behaviour, like hiding the car keys or father's wallet. As with all young children it is advisable to keep an eye on an unoccupied child, particularly if they are extraordinarily quiet.

Discipline, and the teaching of structure and limits, play a key role for a slow learner. A child with Down's syndrome who is not taught to behave is effectively given an additional disadvantage. As with any child in a new environment, after a period of assessment a child with Down's syndrome is likely to 'test' the adults in charge of them. A firm but sympathetic patient response is required. It must be remembered that boredom is a common cause for frequent bad behaviour; it is important to ensure that the work set for the child is adequately stimulating and not underestimating of ability.

To encourage any undesirable behaviour by laughter or smiles when the child is young may lead to later problems that are not so easy to sort out. It is far more important to praise good behaviour frequently than to give attention to misbehaviour. Misbehaviour should be stopped with the minumum of fuss, or even ignored. Criticism and the emphasis of failure merely undermine confidence. These twin strategies – the praising of good behaviour and the ignoring of bad behaviour – are something that should evolve through discussions between parents and teaching staff; inconsistency leaves children confused and poorly behaved.

Hearing and sight

As explained in Chapter 6, many children with Down's syndrome are prone to colds, and the resultant catarrh can invade the Eustachian tube (leading from the throat to the middle ear) and temporarily affect hearing. If parents or staff suspect such a hearing loss, a full assessment should be obtained. Hearing loss may make learning even more difficult and delay the development of language concepts.

If a child has to wear a hearing aid they will undoubtedly need help with it at school, and this ought to be explained to the staff. It ought also to be explained that the use of the hearing aid may give rise to a fear or dislike of loud noise.

Many children with Down's syndrome need to wear glasses, and these should be chosen to suit the child's individual facial features. One aspect of Down's syndrome is a small bridge to the nose, which means that glasses tend to slip down and become a nuisance rather than useful. Glasses frames less likely to slip are available, with different bridge and longer ear pieces. Contact lenses are a successful alternative in many, but need careful supervision.

Teachers should check that the child arrives each day with the glasses and departs with them at the end of each session. Teachers need to know if a child needs assistance in using the glasses, and whether they need to be used all the time or only for close work. The glasses should also be checked after meals to see if they need cleaning.

The eyes of a child with Down's syndrome may not adapt quickly from bright light to shadow. This can cause the child to trip on unseen steps, or on uneven floors. Staff should be aware that a child with poor sight should be allowed to hold a book wherever is found to be most convenient, even if it is rather close to the eyes, or tilted.

Finally if a child is sight or hearing impaired, they will need to be able to see their teacher's face. A central position near the front is ideal, avoiding being placed facing a window or any other bright source of light.

Physical activities and health

As explained earlier, children with Down's syndrome have lower muscle tone than other children, and this can give rise to problems with coordination and gait. In particular, the slack hip muscles can mean that physical activity is difficult. Because of this, extra encouragement and help may be needed for the child to achieve exercises involving hopping, skipping, running, climbing, kicking and balancing. This may give rise to frustration in team games and sport at times, but the children should never be discouraged from joining in. Other children tend to be good coaches, and swimming, dancing, PE and games will all help with muscle tone, general fitness and coordination. Participation should always be encouraged and achievement praised.

At meal times it should be remembered that a child with

Children with Down's syndrome enjoy the same activities as others.

Down's syndrome often has an excellent appetite but may be prone to excess weight gain. Obesity can cause serious problems. Kind dinner-ladies have been known to get great delight from seeing third helpings disappear with great voracity, but they need appropriate advice. A good diet is to be encouraged, in addition to exercise, and refined sugars avoided in sweets and drinks.

Poor coordination of the muscles of chewing and swallowing may cause a child with Down's syndrome to eat slowly. This needs bringing to the attention of the staff, so that extra time can be allowed and food chewed properly.

At break-time in cold weather children with Down's syndrome often need slightly more attention than usual (advice to put on or take off a pullover or coat) because of their poor temperature control and vulnerable skin.

With appropriate preparation, attending nursery and later school is an enjoyable experience for all children. They have their first taste of social independence and have many new learning experiences. Parents see their toddlers emerging as young children ready to take on the next important and exciting developmental steps.

8

Progress at school

Children with Down's syndrome can learn a great deal, especially when emphasis is placed on praise and confidence building. Gold stars or ticks on a chart as rewards for achievement, linked with a system of simple treats, is often effective. If a reward system such as this is being used at home to encourage a particular developmental step such as potty training, it is entirely appropriate that the same system is used at school too. This can usually be achieved after appropriate discussion with the staff. All of us respond to praise, and it is worth remembering to speak only good of a child when in earshot; children will want to live up to the expectations of the adults they like, and may well understand much more of what is being said than the adults give them credit for. The positive term 'special needs' is preferable to a negative term like handicapped.

Communication between home and school is obviously vital with any child, and is to be valued. Parents might want to watch a school's TV programme so that discussions about the programme can go on at home with the child. This will help them build a greater understanding of what they have seen. By following up what is happening at school, parents can help children practise and reinforce new skills. If a home/school book is introduced, it should be used in conjunction with personal contact wherever possible.

Differences in school-based 'academic' ability between children with Down's syndrome and other children become more apparent from the later part of infant school onwards. Every encouragement and opportunity for a child to progress should be given. Some things to think of follow:

- Children with Down's syndrome do not always initiate the learning process; if progress is not being made, teachers should identify which step the child needs to learn next.

- The child's grasp of each new step should be checked.
- It might help to teach simple wording which the child can gradually learn to repeat as an accompaniment to their actions; for example, 'Hold, over and push through' for doing up buttons.
- One cannot assume that the child will understand such basic terms as 'top of the page', 'first', 'last', 'a lot', 'more' (in the mathematical sense); the child's comprehension might lead to a very literal interpretation.

Comprehension and speech will not be at the same level as other children. Every task therefore will need to be broken down and taught in the smallest possible steps, perhaps starting with the last stage; for example the child should start with the task of sliding the last piece of a jigsaw puzzle into place, with some gentle help if necessary. Enormous satisfaction will then be gained by having completed the task. These methods can be used at home as well for tasks such as dressing. For example, children can be taught how to put on trousers by teaching them the last step first.

This principle of breaking things down into simple steps might have to be applied even to routine instructions. For instance a child with Down's syndrome might be confused by being told 'Come and show me your picture, you will need to bring your book and pencil too'. It would be more helpful to break it down into a sequence: 'Pick up your book. Now pick up your pencil. Bring them to me. Now show me your picture'.

Staff should be wary of assuming that the child has understood a step in the task that might seem obvious to others; for example if your child is being taken horse-riding, it ought to be explained to them that the horse is alive and likes to be petted before they attempt to climb on its back.

Bearing in mind that some children with Down's syndrome have short stature, consideration should be given to whether the height of activities, such as sand and water trays, will need to be adjusted or whether the child will need to stand on a block. It is always worth bearing in mind that it is often the least able children in a group who end up with the least efficient equipment – for example, bent scissors, or an underinflated ball – which further hampers progress.

Speech and language

Children with Down's syndrome often have delayed speech, their language skills being fairly consistently slower to develop than other motor and cognitive skills. Much help and encouragement can be given in this area, and the child will certainly benefit from being amongst other more talkative children.

Part of the problem is slowness to develop concepts of language. Communication begins at birth, and parents soon begin to recognise the hungry or tired cry. Good eye contact is established by three months, by which time most babies will be returning smiles and establishing the long-lasting relationship with their parents. It is within this framework of loving parent–child interaction that communication skills develop. At first these will involve changing facial expressions, gesture and tone of voice. Later the children, by this time in the second or third year, will begin to associate particular patterns of sound with particular situations and by so doing work out the meaning of words. The children will then be able to attempt the sounds themselves, at first unclearly but later more expertly.

The next step is putting ideas and therefore words together in short phrases. Gradually the building blocks of spoken language come together and the use of language begins to blossom. Children with Down's syndrome, however, continue to show difficulty in learning the rules of grammar, which slows further development. As they hear sentences which are more complicated, their relatively poor auditory sequential memory also puts them at a disadvantage to children of the same mental age, for it is the auditory sequential memory that helps us to recall what we have heard and in what order. Clearly, this is very important in allowing the brain to decode the sound it receives and attribute meaning to it.

Table showing the rate of acquisition of language skills in Down's syndrome				
Activity	Children with DS		Normal children	
	Average age month	Range month	Average age month	Range month
Reacts to sounds	1	½–1½		0–1
Turns to sound of voice	7	4–8	4	2–6
Say da-da-, ma-ma	11	7–18	8	5–14
Responds to familiar words	13	10–18	8	5–14
Responds to simple verbal instruction	16	12–24	10	6–14
Jabbers expressively	18	12–30	12	9–18
Says first word(s)	18	13–36	14	10–23
Shows needs by gesture	22	14–30	14½	11–19
A few two-word sentences	30	18–60+		
Uses words spontaneously and to communicate	1½–6 years			

Cunningham (1982).

Another part of the problem is poor coordination of the speech muscles, which, like other muscles in the body, are affected by the motor dyspraxia in Down's syndrome (see Chapter 6). Exercising these muscles can be useful:

- Games which make use of speech sounds can be played to good value, for example 'p,p,p' copies the noise a small motor boat makes, 's,s,s' the sound of a snake.
- Blowing and sucking games also strengthen the mouth muscles.
- Playing with a toy telephone will develop the use of, and familiarity with, speech.
- Repeating of nursery rhymes will gradually increase fluency and accustom the child to the natural rhythms of speech.

The effect a large tongue might have on speech development

has probably been overemphasised in the past. Efforts to teach the child to keep the tongue inside the mouth are usually successful, although patience is needed. At school a secret sign, direct to the child, could be employed by the staff, while at home it could be turned into a game, or reminders used, such as stroking downwards under a child's chin. All the exercises mentioned in this section will gradually increase the child's mouth and tongue control and improve articulation.

If it is felt that a child is seriously frustrated by not being able to communicate by talking it is often possible for them to learn Makaton sign language. This can be achieved at quite an early age, often from the second year of life onwards. If the signs are used together with speech, the development of language concepts is encouraged and a lot of frustration through non-communication avoided.

The child who enjoys books is the one most likely to have least trouble recognising pictures and later words. Teachers may be surprised to learn that teaching a child with Down's syndrome to read also improves their language concepts and therefore speech. In some children with Down's syndrome it might not be necessary for them to complete the course of pre-reading skills before going on to read; whether or not this is the case will require discussion with the teacher. However, as with all children, final success in reading varies greatly in children with Down's syndrome.

Once the child can recognise his or her name when it is written down, words can be introduced progressively until, eventually, sentences can be read. In all relevant activities – drawing for example – the child should be encouraged to work from left to right as a preparation for reading and writing.

It should be borne in mind that extra patience on the part of listeners may be needed when the child is trying to speak. Expressive language is of vital importance to any child, and nothing is more frustrating than not being able to put ideas and points of view to other people. Great patience is required to ensure that a language-impaired child is not discouraged from attempting to speak. Staff should always listen carefully, and ensure that the child is given plenty of opportunity to attempt to answer questions and join in discussion. It takes a while for children with Down's syndrome to find the confidence to put their ideas into words, so it helps if the rest of the

Most children with Down's syndrome will be able to read and write when they are older. They should be encouraged to explore books when younger.

group or class are encouraged to be patient. After a while teachers get much better insight into a child's attempts at speaking, and very soon become just as good as the child's parents at understanding what is being said.

Having said that, a high proportion of adults with Down's syndrome have difficulty in making themselves understood by strangers, and about 40 per cent have stammering or stuttering as a symptom. Relaxation techniques and speech therapy advice may help, but it is not yet clear whether this symptom improves in time as it does in younger people who do not have Down's syndrome.

The intelligibility of the speech of adolescents with Down's syndrome				
	Girls		Boys	
	Under 14	Over 14	Under 14	Over 14
Parents usually understand	88%	86%	86%	73%
Strangers usually understand	45%	32%	10%	18%

(From Buckley & Sacks 1986)

With the advent of modern technology, far more teaching opportunities and communication aids are becoming available to people with continuing communication difficulties. This technology, however, cannot really match the value of a language-rich environment and the loving encouragement of parents and interested teachers.

Dexterity

Limited dexterity and coordination is frequently a problem for children with Down's syndrome when they first go to school or playschool, and it may be some years before the child can give attention to two separate activities at once – for example, walk and put on a pair of gloves at the same time, or talk and eat. However, this is often what is expected at school, for example using one hand to steady some bricks while the other hand is used to add further bricks to the structure. Some

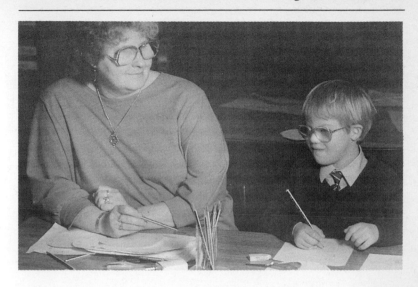

Drawing and cutting out – to encourage fine motor skills.

approaches that may be useful in encouraging dexterity are as follows:

- A reminder of which hand to use – children with Down's syndrome can get confused about which their dominant hand is.
- The fingers of a child with Down's syndrome are often short and the thumbs set low, making it difficult to hold a pen or pencil. Use of the fingers and thumbs can be improved by playing games that require the child to pick up small objects, perhaps from a narrow-topped container using only the finger and thumbs.
- Finger-game rhymes will also help strengthen the fingers and encourage them to move individually.
  – Fine control of the fingers is not possible for a seated child whose feet are dangling. A child with short legs, like a child with Down's syndrome, benefits from the provision of a foot rest.
- Scissors are best controlled if they are held with the forefinger along the shaft and the second or third finger in

the lower finger-hold.
- If buttons are difficult the problem can be eased by resewing the buttons on with a longer shank.
- Exercises in drama and games can be used to increase and improve hand-eye coordination.

Children with Down's syndrome will need plenty of encouragement with fine motor skills, and in particular with writing. Despite the fact that pencil control might be poor, if writing is taught carefully from the start, with emphasis on correctly formed letters, much can be achieved. Because of the relationship between the fingers and thumb, a child with Down's syndrome often grips the pen or pencil in a different way (in the mid-hand rather than the knuckle) and this can cause additional problems.

Concentration

Children with Down's syndrome often have limited concentration for some activities. If pictures are used in teaching, for example, they should not be cluttered up with misleading material, particularly when counting. A change of activity may produce a better response.

The attention span of some children with Down's syndrome is also fairly short. Encouraging the child gradually to spend a little longer at activities will help to extend the concentration span, albeit slowly. If a child shows reluctance to progress from the knowledge that has been assimilated to attempt something new it could well indicate that they have come up against a concept for which they are not ready. By practising their schoolwork and becoming more confident in their own abilities, skills will become consolidated, putting them in a better position to progress to the next stage. It will often be necessary for teachers to devise new and more interesting ways to achieve this repetition. Other children in the class may be able to help in this respect and benefit by practising their own skills at the same time.

Recreation and break-times

Much has been said about the importance of free play at break-times and lunchtimes for schoolchildren, in that they give them a chance to get away from the structure and discipline, however creative it might be in the classroom. But these breaks are not always so helpful or enjoyable for the child with Down's syndrome, who can often be left rather isolated and away from their more socially able and articulate peers.

In such an unstructured situation a child can become vulnerable and may unwittingly become involved in unacceptable activities. Staff can help to a certain extent by exerting efforts to ensure that children with Down's syndrome do become involved in the games of others. However, it can be disadvantageous to press the point too far, and it is sometimes equally advantageous for the teaching assistants involved to take the children with special needs to one side during the long breaks and engage them in different activities suitable for their own ability.

Today's child

Today children with Down's syndrome have a very different lot to that of their counterparts of 15, or even 10, years ago. They are very much part of the family and society in which they live. They expect to join in when encouraged, to explore given the opportunity, and to develop into participating members of society. We owe it to every child to help them reach their full potential.

Down's syndrome is no more than a probability statement. There is a wide range of ability, and academic skills are not to be confused with social skills. Integration brings the advantage that children may learn about disability from an early age; children with learning difficulties follow their peers' example and feel peer pressure. Adequate support is essential. An educational placement is appropriate when a child is happy in school, learning steadily and not disruptive. Where difficulties arise, the support level and placement need review.

9

Growing up and adult life

This chapter will look at the growing opportunities for people with Down's syndrome as they reach adulthood. Medical, social and legal aspects will all be examined.

Life expectancy

It is now clear that the life expectancy of people with Down's syndrome is greater than previously believed. Institutional life no doubt led to less than optimal care in some cases, and exaggerated the risk of infectious diseases being passed from one to another. Now that people with Down's syndrome are brought up and live in the community, there is a far more optimistic outlook.

The major determinant of mortality in the first three decades, and particularly in the first year, of life is the presence of congenital heart disease. Over 90 per cent of children without a heart problem survive the first year, whereas about 25 per cent of those with congenital heart disease will die in infancy. A recent study from British Columbia reviewed the life expectancy of 1,341 people with Down's syndrome; for those with congenital heart disease survival to age 5 was 62 per cent, to age 10 was 57 per cent, to age 20 was 53 per cent, and to 30 was 50 per cent. For those without congenital heart anomalies the corresponding figures showed survival to age 5 in 87 per cent, to age 10 in 85 per cent, to age 20 in 82 per cent and to 30 in 79 per cent.

Disordered immunity still accounts for a number of early deaths, and after the age of 40 the emergence of Alzheimer's disease tends to give a life expectancy less than that expected with other mentally disabling conditions. A study based at Stoke Park Hospital, in Bristol, between 1976 and 1980 showed the average life expectancy of people with Down's syndrome was 55 for men and 53 for women. Clearly when plans are being drawn up for financial provision, social support and housing of people with Down's syndrome, these sort of statistics need bearing in mind.

Biological maturation

Information on the physical and sexual maturation of adolescents with Down's syndrome is limited, and until recently has largely been on those living in institutional care, where reported abnormalities seemed common. More recent studies have been on home-reared children, with fewer abnormalities being seen.

Biological maturation in males with Down's syndrome

The development of secondary sexual characteristics (those that appear at puberty) in males with Down's syndrome is essentially the same as that in the general population. There is normal development of pubic hair, but beard growth is on the whole slower than in the general population. There is a tendency for testicular size to be smaller, but many men with Down's syndrome have normally-sized testicles. Similarly, stretched penile length tends to be shorter.

Early studies may have overestimated the prevalence of genital abnormalities in boys. The previously quoted incidence of undescended testicles has been as high as 50 per cent. One recent study of home-reared children with Down's syndrome from Maryland showed two of 53 to have perineal hypospadias (where the urinary opening is not at the end of the penis but at its base), two with bilaterally undescended testicles, and five with retractile testicles. These findings are probably more representative of the actual prevalence.

Study of endocrine function has also shown conflicting results. Plasma testosterone (the sex hormone leading to masculine features) has on the whole been shown to be normal, but a number of studies have shown a significant number of boys to have raised levels of follicle stimulating hormone and luteinising hormone. These two hormones are produced by the pituitary gland, follicle stimulating hormone stimulating sperm production. These results are found before and after puberty, and suggest a partial primary gonadal dysfunction. Studies suggest that this may progress with age, and degenerative change has been seen in some testes examined histologically. There may be inefficient feedback between the gonads and the hypothalamic–pituitary axis (the way the gonad and brain interact to secure normal hormone levels) or a lack of target organ response to circulating stimulating hormone (page 61). The disordered membrane function referred to in the chapter on biochemical genetics is probably also important in this respect.

Data on spermatogenesis (sperm production by the testes) are limited because of the problems of sperm collection for laboratory study. It does appear that there is reduced fertility in a high proportion of males with Down's syndrome. Where sperm counts are normal, motility is often poor and the proportion of abnormal forms high. Nevertheless, males with Down's syndrome cannot be assumed to be sterile; 1990 saw the first report of a pregnancy where the father was confirmed to be a man with Down's syndrome.

Biological maturation in females with Down's syndrome

The development of secondary sexual characteristics in females is the same as in the general population, although there are reports of axillary (armpit) hair in females being lost at a relatively early age and a relative lack of apocrine (sweat) glands in the axilla.

Although the onset of menstruation is a little delayed in Down's syndrome, it is by no more than a few months, and the differences are unimportant. In other respects the characteristics of the menstrual cycle are the same as for all women.

Whether ovulation occurs is more difficult to establish. Studies seem to show that about a third of women with Down's syndrome show a definite pattern of ovulation, a third no evidence of ovulation and in about a third the evidence is indeterminate.

The number of reported cases of pregnancy in women with Down's syndrome is strikingly low. To date there have been 30 reported pregnancies occurring in 26 women. Hormonal studies show the same elevated serum levels of FSH and LH as in men, implying a similar primary gonadal disfunction.

Self-esteem

Adolescence should not only be a time for physical development, but also one for emotional maturation. Disabled children are more vulnerable to a variety of psycho-social problems, and parents and carers need to be aware of this so that they may encourage confidence and independence rather than reinforcing a sense of separateness and the need constantly to rely on others.

From quite an early age children with Down's syndrome will be aware that they are different in many ways from other children. This sense of isolation may be seen for the first time when children enter nursery school and feel the pressure of children the same age as themselves communicating freely and generally performing more adeptly. After a while they may become aware or perceive that their peers are having negative feelings towards them. The fact others react in this way may lead to feelings of hurt. Through this exposure to other people outside the immediate family, children with Down's syndrome gradually perceive that others consider them to be different and inferior. Security comes from a feeling of belonging and being similar to others; when these feelings are absent the effect can be devastating on the individual.

Within society there is a considerable tolerance of disability, but beneath the surface there is often an involuntary revulsion at the problem. (It is this revulsion that first confronts parents following the birth of their child with Down's syndrome.) The expression of these mixed emotions can be confusing. At times children with Down's syndrome may be subjected to overt kindness; at other times to frank embarrassment.

Negative attitudes towards disabled people have been shown to increase with age in children. When they are very young they do not mind playing with disabled children, but as they grow older they slowly show a greater intolerance. This is because of the essential part of growing up already referred to: that of a feeling of similarity with one's peers; to be seen to befriend a disabled child may be seen as socially disadvantageous in a peer group. Gradually as they get older children with Down's syndrome realise they are being avoided because of their disability. This gradual growth of awareness of society's norms unfortunately often leads to feelings of self-rejection. The inability to change the impairment leads to feelings of inferiority, the self-image to alter and self-esteem to fall. With increasing maturity young people with Down's syndrome can even start to assume that they are disabled because they have done something wrong, which in turn can lead to feelings of guilt.

Parents have a central role in promoting independence and confidence in their children. Overprotectiveness can lead to infantilisation (persistently treating a child like a baby) and to problems with self-help, self-reliance and inadequacy. Worse, if parents show themselves to be embarrassed or to reject their children in company, the child with Down's syndrome will have additional problems with self-esteem, feeling the parents have been failed. These thoughts can lead in turn to social isolation and depression, with an ultimate detrimental effect on performance.

Parents need to show warmth and sympathetic support, tempered by firmness when their child shrinks from a task they are probably capable of. They should talk to their child about their difficulties and this should reduce tension. The children themselves, where possible, should be encouraged to talk to others about this too. This can reduce discomfort, anxiety and uncertainty when new friendships are being made and new situations being entered. It minimises the chance of subtle or overt rejection by others. Ability should be emphasised rather than disability, and a balance should be struck in life where enjoyable tasks should be pursued in order to balance those things a child finds difficult.

Doctors can be guilty of showing disproportionate attention to purely medical aspects of a child's condition, whilst ignoring the psycho-social consequences. It is these aspects of a child's life that may prove to be the most disadvantageous, and to maintain good standards of medical care they need to be addressed.

Friendships

Adolescence is usually a time for moving away from the family, increasing independence and creating friendships. However, although teenagers with Down's syndrome have the usual range of teenage interests – pop stars, music and sport – they rarely seem able to pursue these interests outside the home with friends of their own age. Instead they tend to spend their time watching the TV or listening to tapes or records. Most are very dependent on their families for social activity.

Much of this social isolation arises out of poor communication skills. Although the speech in four out of five teenagers with Down's syndrome is easily understood by their family, only 30 per cent of girls and 14 per cent of boys are easily understood by strangers. In one survey, only one in three had a good friend and half the girls and a third of the boys saw their friends less than once a week. This loneliness can lead to the creation of imaginary friends in roughly half of teenagers with Down's syndrome; this pattern of behaviour often being established at quite an early age. Conversations may be held with these fantasy friends. This, along with imaginative play with dolls and similar toys, seems to help the teenagers work out things that are bothering them. It must be understood that although this behaviour is not age appropriate, it does not represent a psychosis – psychotic behaviour is actually very rare in Down's syndrome. Adults can use this play as a cue to help young people with Down's syndrome to overcome some of their worries.

Much can be done to help loneliness and integration by imaginative enterprise on the part of parents to find social outlets outside the home, and by continuing efforts to improve communication skills. For example in Britain, Mencap run Gateway clubs which allow even the more severely disabled an opportunity to socialise with others, some of whom will be more and some less disabled than them. A number of charitable organisations and some local authorities run Outreach clubs where the emphasis is on social integration, with trips to local restaurants or places of interest. Cubs, Brownies, Scouts and Guides all offer places to young people with Down's syndrome, as do many keep-fit and martial arts centres. The Uphill Ski Club was founded with the disabled in mind and many Outward Bound centres run courses for the disabled too.

Success in many of these ventures depends on a 'buddy' system, whereby a more able person will befriend, encourage and support someone with disability. The Ocean Youth Club is a good example of this, where a number of learning disabled people have had an introduction to sailing. In the USA a number of neighbourhood 'buddy' schemes have grown up where this sort of encouragement and support is pursued on a community basis. Both those with and without learning disability voice benefits for the schemes, which often lead to feelings of mutual respect and lasting friendships.

Love and marriage

Sexual awareness and curiosity are delayed in young people with Down's syndrome, and in some never appear. Thoughts of sexuality, whether male or female, seem to remain on a childish level. Well over half adolescents and young adults are interested in the opposite sex, and many have special friends, but the emotional involvement is non-sexual. Emotional ties are warm and loving and the making of new friends is treated with enjoyment. But relationships with the opposite sex rarely go beyond a platonic friendship. Physical contact is common, but often does not go beyond hugging and kissing. The choice of the partner seems to be based on the degree of attention and emotion received in return, rather than physical attraction.

There is far less desire for sexual intercourse than in most people, and sexual activity is usually limited to masturbation. Having said that, in institutional care only about half the young people seem to indulge in self-gratification.

Families may need advice on how to control behaviour perceived by others to be sexual. Children should be taught that masturbation is something to be done in private and that, after a certain age, hugging and kissing as a show of affection is not socially acceptable where strangers are involved.

Some adults with Down's syndrome will of course mature to a degree whereby they can develop a friendship with another person and also have a need for a sexual relationship. A small number of people with Down's syndrome marry, and this number is likely to increase. This sort of development will need a lot of support from family, friends and society. In a changing world it is likely to be seen with ever increasing frequency as appropriate support reaches more people with

Down's syndrome, allowing them to reach their true potential.

Down's syndrome and the law

As people with Down's syndrome achieve better lifestyles for themselves, they will be increasingly expected to make choices, take risks and be responsible for the consequences of personal decisions. Even quite severely impaired people may be able to make simple choices where the issues are explained carefully in appropriate language. The mental impairment, of course, makes them more vulnerable to exploitation by the unscrupulous; they can often be persuaded where biased information is given.

The issue of consent

Many of these issues are particularly pertinent where the issue of sexual activity is concerned. Section 7 of the Sexual Offences Act 1956 states that it is an offence for a man to have unlawful sexual intercourse with a woman who is a 'mental defective', where unlawful means outside marriage, and defective means a person suffering from a state of arrested or incomplete development of mind that includes severe impairment of intelligence and social functioning. It seems unlikely that a woman with Down's syndrome who has severe learning difficulties could ever validly consent to marriage, even if the opportunity arose, so lawful sex in this context seems only possible where the man was himself incapable of realising her state of impairment. As the purpose of this Act is to protect vulnerable women who might be exploited, prosecution would no doubt be pursued only very selectively.

Parents of the more severely learning disabled young women with Down's syndrome are often rightly worried about their daughters' vulnerability to pregnancy, and a number of sterilisations have been carried out for this reason (at least 36 girls under 18 were sterilised in England in 1973 to 1974, and in 1987 the Department of Health stated that around 90 sterilisations were performed each year on women aged under 19). Previously, before proceeding with the sterilisation, medical practitioners would share the particular issues of individual cases with the girl herself, if possible, the girl's parents, social workers and other health care professionals. Under the Mental Health Act 1959, consent could be given on behalf of the individual concerned. This followed the notion that guardianship could be held not only by parents but also by personnel of social services.

The Mental Health Act 1983 replaced this 1959 Act, and significantly restricted the role of guardians in this respect. In particular, they could no longer sign consent forms and this, together with the case of Re B (a minor) heard before the Court of Appeal in 1987, has given learning disabled people a new status in law. Now those with learning difficulties who have enough understanding to give consent to a particular procedure are allowed to do so (previously this was not possible; the guardian had to be asked). Proxy consent is no longer valid in law. This is a welcome development in view of the increasing amount of community care, the rejection of the concept of infantilism and a greater awareness of human rights on the part of people with learning difficulties.

The problem then remains of how to organise the medical care of those who are unable to understand the issues involved. When treatment is not controversial, doctors need to go ahead if possible with the agreement (but not the consent) of parents or usual caretakers of the child. In these circumstances doctors are acting 'in good faith' and showing a 'duty of care'. In an emergency doctors may clearly intervene without the consent of the person involved or the support of close relatives, as the 'principle of necessity' is recognised in law.

The situation gets complicated where the medical procedure involved is of a controversial nature, such as sterilisation. In Re B (a minor) the Court of Appeal authorised an operation to sterilise a mentally handicapped girl of 17. The girl, known as Jeanette, was said to have a mental age of 5 or 6 and to be incapable of understanding the procedure of sterilisation, and therefore not able to give informed consent herself. Lord Justice Dillon said that the Court had jurisdiction to authorise a sterilisation operation on a ward of court (as Jeanette was) in wardship proceedings, but it was a jurisdiction that should be exercised only as a last resort when all other forms of contraception had been considered. It was added that there was no question of a natural parent, or local authority with parental rights, giving consent to a sterilisation operation without first obtaining the leave of the Court.

In reaching its decision the Court had considered an earlier much publicised case, that of Re D (a minor) 1976. This related to an 11-year-old girl with Sotos syndrome who was said to have an IQ of 80 and had a behaviour disorder. Her widowed mother feared that she might become pregnant. Local doctors agreed, but an educational psychologist challenged the appropriateness of this decision. Mrs Justice Heilbron heard that the proposed operation involved the deprivation of a woman's basic human rights to reproduce. Furthermore, if the operation were performed on a woman for non-therapeutic reasons and without her consent, it would be a violation of that right. It was further ruled that such decisions should not be within the doctor's sole clinical judgment, that in the evidence the operation was neither medically indicated nor necessary and would not be in the girl's best interest. Each case would have to be decided by a court on its merits and on the evidence.

In 1989 five law lords found that the 'principle of necessity' should be stretched to controversial situations such as sterilisation. The interpretation is that doctors should act in accordance with a substantial body of medical opinion or be seen to be following the established medical practice of the day so that they might be 'acting in the best interest of the patient'. It is clear from this judgment that when a medical intervention is planned that might be deemed controversial, doctors would be prudent to gain the agreement from a court so that the anticipated controversial intervention 'will not be unlawful'.

At the time of writing the Law Commission and the Department of Health are still investigating the law of consent, and it is to be hoped that rules will soon emerge to guide us all. Recourse to the High Court, the Court of Appeal and thence to the House of Lords is time-consuming, expensive and emotionally draining for the families involved. It is to be hoped that life will become far simpler in this respect. Greater involvement by district health commissions and local ethical committees may well be the way forward.

Meanwhile parents and practitioners are left with some imponderables. If the Court's consent is needed for the sterilisation of a girl with learning difficulties, should it not also be needed for other contraceptive measures? A girl who is incapable of understanding or giving consent to sterilisation is also likely to be incapable of giving informed consent to sexual intercourse or the acceptance of contraception and their side effects. Further legislation and guidance are awaited.

The law and hospitalisation

The Mental Health Act 1983 was an update of previously existing legislation, but unfortunately still confuses the issue of mental illness and learning disability. Where compulsory admission to hospital is concerned the law talks of a central concept of 'mental impairment' (arrested or incomplete development of the mind). Very few people with Down's syndrome are abnormally aggressive or seriously irresponsible, and it is only these who could be compulsorily admitted or detained in hospital because of 'mental disorder', and then it would be for a non-renewable period (maximum 28 days).

Following detention, hospitalisation is for the person's health or safety or for the protection of other people. The admission is for treatment which is designed 'to alleviate or prevent any serious deterioration of the patient's condition'. The patient must be mentally impaired such that hospital care and treatment are appropriate, and it must be impossible to provide this care and treatment elsewhere. A person's nearest relative or an approved social worker can apply for the person's admission, which is based upon two medical recommendations. If the hospital accepts, the patient is detained for up to six months, a period that is then renewable.

In England and Wales doctors can renew a detention order initially for six months and thereafter annually, although this is only if the conditions that were pertinent to the initial admission still apply. However, where the person involved has severe learning difficulties, it must be established that care could not be provided in a different community setting. People can apply to the Mental Health Review Tribunal, which can order the patient to be discharged if the conditions are not fulfilled. When the person involved is not capable of appealing themselves, there is a statutory requirement of hospital managers to apply to the Tribunal on their behalf at three-yearly intervals. With the advent of community care, providing it is adequately resourced, long-term detention of this sort should disappear; hospitalisation should then only be required where 'danger' is involved.

In practice very few people in England are admitted or detained under the provisions of this Act. Where compulsory admission is undertaken, it is usually by use of short-term powers, where the protections for the patients are fewer. The first of these is a 28-day order, where the patient must be suffering from a mental disorder (see above). The conditions for admission are not as stringent as those already considered, but the patient does have a right of appeal within 14 days. A 72-hour order can be used for admission for assessment in an emergency; the same conditions apply, but the agreement of only one doctor is required. Down's syndrome itself does not predispose to conditions that lead to admission of this sort, except under very rare circumstances; this is where mental illness exists alongside the learning disability, and treatment is required as it would be in the general population.

Thankfully most admissions and detentions are through informal admission procedures on a voluntary basis. The problem is that, where learning disability is concerned, the people concerned are vulnerable to suggestion that is not necessarily in their own interest; the naivity of people with learning difficulties can be misused in a deceitful way. In the past there have been many instances of misleading, unfair or even unkind treatment in institutional care. It is likely that these situations will be less prevalent with increasing care in the community. Furthermore, the new regulations reduce the powers of guardianship and this should reduce the burden on local authorities, since they no longer imply a parental role. People with Down's syndrome should now be able to live in a reasonable fashion in the community without too many restrictions upon their freedom and with institutionalisation avoided. Further aspects of the law and people with Down's syndrome are considered in the sections on education and in the next chapter, where the rights to life and to treatment are also considered.

The Children Act 1989 is the most comprehensive piece of legislation enacted about children and replaces the previously fragmented pieces of legislation as a comprehensive statement on the law relating to the care and protection of children. One of the most important principles behind the act is that the welfare of the child is paramount and that children are generally best looked after within their own family. Where other agencies are required to supervise the care of the child it is stated that this is best done in the context of a partnership between those agencies and the family concerned. Much of the act deals with the issue of child protection but important consideration is also given to children with disabilities. It is hoped that the creation of a joint register of disabled children between health, education and social services will greatly facilitate the identification, registration and a co-ordinated provision of services. This applies not only at any early stage when assessments were being drawn up and procedures defined in the 1981 Education Act (see above) but also in relation to the provision of respite care and the subsequent placement of adults with severe learning difficulties in residential community houses.

Integration, education and employment prospects

With the closure of the large long-stay residential hospitals for people with learning difficulties, significant changes are taking place in relation to large sections of the disabled adult community. In the years ahead more and more adults with Down's syndrome will find themselves supported in community houses, either living alone or with a small number of people of similar ability. Even for those adults with Down's syndrome who are less able very sheltered environments or special-care facilities will always be needed, but there is no reason why this should not be provided in the comfort of a small unit with a homely environment rather than in the large Victorian hospitals that achieved little but heightened isolation.

For the more able, greater integration into the community will require further education, particularly in relation to developing independence skills. Currently only about one in six young adults with Down's syndrome go to further education colleges on life-skill courses, but it is likely that this proportion will increase. Given adequate interest on the part of the staff, and adequate resources, much can be achieved, even with the more severely learning disabled.

A good example of this is a study carried out at the Universities of Minnesota and Maryland. The study described how a 16-year-old youth with severe learning difficulties was taught over a six-week period how to use a local bowling alley. Such language as he had was unintelligible, but he was shown how to overcome this problem by the use of cards expressing simple wishes. It was not long before he learnt who he needed to see for appropriate footwear and the bowls, and, after an enjoyable game, how to use the food and drink vending machines. The skills acquired in this setting were clearly useful to the young man in other circumstances too. This shows how if people are imaginative and are not confined by prejudgments, much can be achieved for those with learning difficulties in society.

Currently about 75 per cent of adults with Down's syndrome go to local adult training centres or sheltered workshops. There are advantages to this arrangement; it structures the day for the people involved, and they have an opportunity to develop friendships with people of similar ability. However, the tasks available to them are often rather mundane, and the environment is often not rich enough for many to reach their natural full potential.

It is disappointing to learn that only about 1 per cent of adults with Down's syndrome are in gainful employment. This is far fewer than would be expected if one predicts the potential usefulness of people of their ability. A wide range of unskilled and semi-skilled jobs are within the intellectual competence of most school-leavers with Down's syndrome – kitchen work, gardening, portering are but a few examples. As employees, people with Down's syndrome often prove to be more punctual, reliable and malleable than other people employed in the same type of work.

The acquisition of employment does much to enhance the life of any adult. Apart from structuring the day and improving self-esteem, it enhances income, which in turn brings the opportunity to improve other aspects of life; particularly the opportunity to live alone, or at least with a smaller number of people rather than living communally in a community house. For those from richer families this ideal may be secured through private means, but for most much

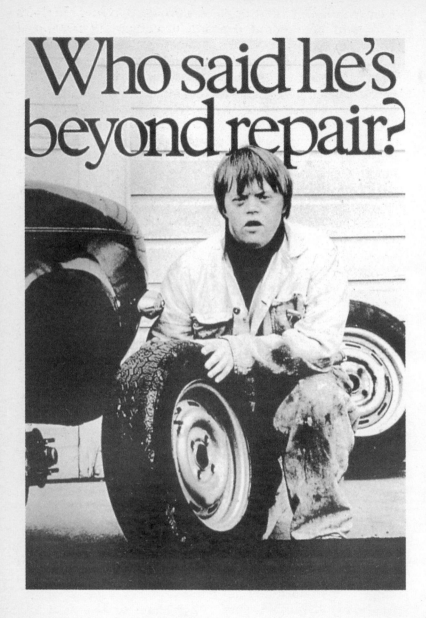

reliance will be placed on local authority facilities. Facilities are very variable from one region to another. The best model for care seems to be for local self-help groups for the disabled to liaise with local and education authorities so that duplication of effort is avoided. In so doing young adults with Down's syndrome must be encouraged to speak for themselves and to achieve a degree of self-determination. Key workers are allocated to individual families and the quagmire of undue bureaucracy is simplified. It is likely that in the future we shall see the inadequate resources allocated by central government funds bolstered by funds raised in the charitable and private sector. If the final result is better facilities for our adult learning disabled population then nothing should be placed in the way of this development.

In summary, it can be said that the last few decades have brought greater acknowledgment of the need for self-determination of people with learning disabilities. The next few decades will see the fulfilment of that ideal, with a greater number living independently in the community, with access to work appropriate to their level of ability, which in turn will secure an enhancement of the quality of their lives.

Changes of this sort require extra resources and careful preparation. Sadly many local authorities have been under-resourced in this respect. Now that a much better pattern of community care has been defined it is to be hoped the political will is retained to achieve it.

10

Hopes and fears

Birth and the right to life

A number of children with Down's syndrome are born with life-threatening conditions, some remediable and some irremediable. Where the problem cannot be helped, adequate support for the family and good nursing care is what is required.

When a baby with Down's syndrome is born with a remediable medical problem, such as certain heart conditions or duodenal atresia, a potential area of conflict between parents and health care professionals arises. The medical and nursing staff have a duty to remedy the problem and preserve life. The parents may see this as their 'way out', confronted as they are by their initial sense of revulsion and a fear of what the future holds for them. The thought that the problem might be allowed to go away holds some attraction. They are already in the throes of grieving for the child who did not arrive, and the thought that nature might actually relieve them of the problem before it has become burdensome can be quite comforting.

At times in the past doctors have held much sympathy with the feelings of parents in this situation, to the point where they have allowed children to die, or even secured a child's death by means of sedation. The doctors have shared the revulsion and abhorrence of the thought of parents having to cope with the handicap, and have also held a view that they are perhaps saving the children themselves some unhappiness, if not suffering, by securing their demise. The sedated babies failed to demand feeds and died within a few days of birth.

In recent years a consultant paediatrician was charged with murder (R. v. Arthur) in circumstances similar to these. In the course of the trial the charge was replaced by one of attempted murder as more forensic evidence was submitted, and ultimately the defendant was found not guilty. Although the trial left many important legal and ethical principles unaddressed, it did make it clear that juries are quite disinclined to find doctors guilty of murder in these circumstances. More recently still (Re C, a minor), a judge found that it would be 'not unlawful' to let a child die where severe disability existed and where suffering would be avoided.

Whereas there are many situations in medicine where it can readily be seen that to prolong life would be wrong in terms of common ethics and humanity, the diagnosis of Down's syndrome alone at birth could never justify this. At this stage future development cannot be predicted. Most parents would be able to hope for a child who at worst would have a moderate learning disability. As we have seen already, this allows many the potential to gain at least some independence in life, employment, and to find a degree of satisfaction and contentment.

This is a time when parents should be able to expect great sensitivity and good counselling skills on the part of doctors and others in attendance. If curative surgery is to be undertaken, they need good information presented in a simple and readily understandable way on the future prospect of their child. They also need guidance on the reasons behind the feelings they are experiencing; through insight of this kind they can begin to support each other. As a last resort doctors may turn to the law so that the child can be made a ward of court to minimise any delay of the curative surgery.

Unfortunately, the model of good practice outlined above has not always been apparent. Doctors' attitudes have been studied by David Silverman, working in a British paediatric cardiology clinic in the early 1980s. Using only a small sample, he highlighted a number of revealing issues. For example, in 10 consultations with parents of children with Down's syndrome, on not one occasion did the cardiologist ask 'Is he/she well?' In the 22 control families, 11 were greeted with this question. The inference here is that the physician made the assumption that a child with Down's syndrome could not be well and therefore did not bother to ask. It was also noted that, when the statement of diagnosis was made, in 75 per cent of the control families the anatomical description of the heart defect was tempered with some statement of reassurance. Acknowledging that the heart defects in Down's syndrome might have been relatively more severe, it is noteworthy that in only one of 12 families studied at the diagnostic stage was there any such supportive statement. In the words of Silverman, many doctors seem to perceive that 'a child who is not altogether whole or is imperfect may turn out to be imperfectable'. In other words, the misunderstandings some doctors have about Down's syndrome may influence them when they are thinking about treatment, and some children might not get the treatment they deserve.

Doctors may also tend to discuss illnesses or problems identified by parents as 'just Down's syndrome' or 'typically Down's syndrome'. If not pursued, the lack of further investigation or follow-up can have serious consequences for development or health.

Previous authors have shown that medical judgment about mental ability in children with Down's syndrome made doctors predisposed not to intervene in congenital heart disease unless parents were actively in favour; for example, they were much more likely to operate upon a given heart condition where the child had a urogenital anomaly as opposed to Down's syndrome. Such prejudgment also exists in other areas. Doctors visiting families at home to decide on entitlement to attendance allowance often assure the family of success (because their child has Down's syndrome) before any assessment of the child involved has actually taken place. This no longer should arise, as attendance allowance is awardable from birth, a time at which assessment of most children and how their future demands will differ from the norm is impossible. Medical practitioners should not mix in their minds the concepts of health and handicap.

Reference has already been made to SCOPE's 'Right from the Start' campaign (page 36). It is hoped that as the medical and nursing professions learn more about how to introduce families to the idea that their child has a learning disability, doctors and nurses themselves will learn more of how to influence society to lessen the disadvantage of the condition.

Specific therapies for Down's syndrome

Pseudo-scientific vitamin regimes and intensive developmental programmes share a number of things in common. They are often presented to parents along with a grain of scientific truth, leading them to believe that they might actually represent a rational approach to therapy. The ideas that a vitamin concoction can radically alter body chemistry and that intensive stimulation can make brain cells grow both, on the face of it, seem tenable to the lay person. If one adds to this the ingredients of desperation, gullibility and a magical belief in the healing powers of health care professionals, then it is clear to see why some parents follow this course of action. Even though they may be told that scientific studies fail to show any benefit for the methods they are pursuing, they continue to pursue them because they want to feel they are doing something.

Meanwhile parents will find a variety of practitioners willing to advocate treatment of unproven value, often at some expense. Those involved are very vulnerable to this sort of suggestion. They may not have fully accepted the handicap and yearn to put the problem right. Feelings of guilt may lead them to pursue any opportunity, no matter how spurious the treatment being offered. There is a whole series of anecdotal treatments from centres throughout the world propounded by a very small number of medical practitioners, paramedical practitioners, hypnotists, allergists, reflexologists and cell therapists, whose claims are at best intellectually dishonest, but possibly fraudulent.

Turkel advocates megavitamins for the problem, and there have been a number of exponents of this view. The approach is illogical because children with Down's syndrome have an increased gene dosage effect and vitamins only succeed by acting as co-enzymes, thus driving deficient rather than over-efficient enzyme systems. Long-term toxic effects of some vitamins, notably pyridoxine, vitamin B6, which causes a neuropathy, are documented. Where carefully controlled trials have been carried out, no benefit for this therapy has ever been shown.

Pauling was involved in some of the early studies of what has become known as orthomolecular medicine. He defined this as the treatment 'of mental disorders by the provision of the optimum molecular environment for the mind, especially the optimum concentration of substances normally present in the human body'. In the world of Down's syndrome, Harrell and colleagues (1981) published data on Turkel's 'U' series in

1964, indicating that vitamins enhanced the development of people with Down's syndrome. It must be said, though, that the choice of controls was poor and the work has proved to be unrepeatable.

Bennett and colleagues from Seattle (1983) carried out a randomised control trial of vitamin therapy versus placebo in 20 children with Down's syndrome aged between 5 and 13 years. The study subjects were matched for age, sex, race and socio-economic status. Over the eight-month period of the study no differences in the tested areas were found for development, behaviour, IQ, school achievement, speech and language or neuromotor function. Appearance, growth and health were also the same for the two groups. In the same year Smith and colleagues from Chicago, again using megadoses of vitamins, did a double-blind trial on 45 school-age children, again well matched for controls for measured intelligence, sex, age and home and school environmental characteristics. They were assessed at baseline and after four and eight months, but no differences were seen on the measured variables.

Corman and colleagues carried out a double-blind study of vitamin B6 in infants with Down's syndrome. The rationale for their study resulted from an earlier observation that children with Down's syndrome had a significantly low level of 5-hydroxy-tryptamine (5HT). Administration of 5HT had led to the development of infantile spasms in one in six children so treated. Vitamin B6 is a co-enzyme in the second step of 5HT metabolism. Included in the complex is pyridoxal-5-phosphate, which is a major metabolite involved in the metabolism of brain amino acids, lipid nucleic acids and glycogen metabolism. It is mooted that the reduction in phospholipid content of myelin in Down's syndrome may be due to a relative deficiency of B6. The double-blind part of the study involved 19 infants of less than eight weeks of age. The treated group responded by having significantly elevated levels of 5HT, but this was only sustained during the first year of life. Growth rates, including head circumference, were exactly the same in the two groups at 2 years, as was all psychological testing. However, at 6 years the treated group had a significantly higher social quotient. This aspect of the work has not been repeated. In the open part of the study, where additional people with Down's syndrome were given

B6, a number of them developed significant side-effects, blistering on exposure to sun, vomiting and the emergence of peripheral neuropathy being among the more serious. The peripheral neuropathy well reported in other contexts emerged after about four years' treatment. This illustrates well how the assumption cannot be that vitamins can do no harm. Any therapy used in Down's syndrome stands an equal chance of doing harm as possibly doing some good. Bumbalo and colleagues (1964) and Rowland and Spiker (1985) have also failed to show benefit utilising double-blind procedures for nutritional treatment in Down's syndrome.

Advocates of so-called neurotransmitter therapy fail to acknowledge that the substances are probably not absorbed in their original form, and are therefore pharmacologically useless. Deanol (2-dimethylaminoethanol) is the substance usually mentioned by advocates of 'neurotransmitter therapy'. Deanol may be a precursor of acetylcholine; it has been claimed to enhance cholinergic activity. However, to claim this as its mode of action is purely speculative. The drug has been used in behaviour disorders and has been shown to improve performance in behaviourally disturbed children. Its effect is probably as a central stimulant, much the same as methylphenidate (Ritalin). These drugs carry the disadvantage that they are addictive, and can induce seizures. Ritalin might be considered very rarely for a child with Down's syndrome who has a particularly poor attention span and uncontrollable hyperactivity. Specialist advice is needed, and the drug is probably best used in a double-blind way alongside a placebo so that a good opinion may be formed on whether it is actually helping or not.

Cell therapy, equally, carries no logical rationale. Cell therapy originated in Europe and involves the injection of dried animal foetal cells on a five to six monthly basis. This is, however, rarely done in isolation, and advocates of the therapy usually combine it with a number of pharmacological preparations including vitamins, minerals and thyroid therapy. Randomised double-blind controlled trials are difficult to carry out in these circumstances, where procedures are controversial, intrusive or potentially dangerous, but Foreman and Ward, working at Macquarie University, New South Wales, in Australia, have bravely tried. They compared two groups, one receiving and one not receiving cell therapy plus its associated medication. They placed a newsletter in the National Cell Therapy Association's magazine in Australia, and by this means identified 57 families receiving the therapy, of whom 53 were studied. Controls were matched for age and sex. No differences were found between the two groups in relation to growth, physical appearance including skin and hair, nor on developmental quotients, save for the performance subscale of the Griffiths developmental scale for older children. The observed differences were significant but unimportant and, due to the study design, could well have been determined by confounding variables rather than treatment differences. Their study serves to show that where study groups are small the play of chance may serve to exaggerate or even underestimate the differences between groups. For example, taking the younger children as a whole on the performance scale, the mean score for treated children was 63.9 (SD 14.8) whereas that for controls was 77.1 (SD 16.3). This difference is not significant at the 5 per cent level. However, for older children the performance score for treated children was 57.5 (SD 13.0), whereas that for controls was 46.9 (SD 12.1). This difference is significant at the 5 per cent level but the effect is in the opposite direction to that seen in the younger child. Rather than the treatment having any real effect, a more likely conclusion is that chance has intervened to produce what is likely to be an unrepeatable result.

Piracetum is a drug which has received attention in recent years. In a controlled trial it was shown to improve the performance of children with specific learning difficulties. The advantage noted in the study was significant, measurable but in the classroom setting, arguably anyway, not all that important. The study has not been repeated and substantiated. It is, therefore, premature to suggest that the drug would be of benefit to young people with Down's syndrome. Further studies are required.

Facial plastic surgery

Since the early 1970s facial plastic surgery has been performed on many children with Down's syndrome, hoping to 'normalise' the child's appearance, thus leading to better acceptance by society. Further objectives are to reduce drooling, facilitate better chewing and swallowing, and reduce the frequency of upper respiratory infections. Claims for the improvement of language development, cognitive function, social development and integration are also made. It must be noted, however, that 90 per cent of children with DS do not drool, 85 per cent do not have significant difficulties with eating or chewing and three-quarters of parents feel that their child's facial features do not affect their social development in any negative way.

Partial glossectomy (removal of part of the tongue), lateral canthoplasty (refashioning the shape of the eyes) and enhancement of the zygoma (cheek bone) have all been advocated and carried out. Infection, the wound breaking down and foreshortening of the tongue have all been reported as complications, and time spent in hospital can unsettle children. Controlled assessment of the procedures has failed to show any overall benefit in appearance or articulatory ability.

It must be acknowledged that there may be pressing indications for plastic surgery in a very small number of children with Down's syndrome. Meanwhile, it would seem equally important to pay attention to a child's appearance, dress sense and general hygiene so that acceptance by and integration into society might be achieved.

Early intervention/intensive stimulation

Early intervention programmes are based on the premise that significant improvement in long-term developmental outcome can be achieved by ordered stimulation. Some have made claims that the stimulation actually leads to an increase in nerve cells. This claim is unsubstantiated, but there is animal work that infers that the developing brain hemispheres may retain a degree of plasticity if exposed to new stimuli. What is well established is that intervention programmes can help by offering psychological and social support to the families involved. Through help with adjustment, an environment is created in which opportunity and encouragement help children to reach their full potential.

There have been relatively few scientific evaluations of the benefit of intervention programmes. Studies have shown conflicting results, with benefit shown in some and none in others.

Ludlow and Allen studied home-reared children who did, or did not, receive an intervention programme and compared them with institutionalised children. The children on the intervention programme did best of all, with significantly less decline in developmental quotient beyond the age of 3, and better performance following school entry. This was not, however, a randomised trial, and controls were not matched. In any study comparing developmental outcome it is essential to take note of variables such as number of siblings, socio-economic status and educational level of parents, as these are known to have a strong bearing on developmental attainment.

The work of Cunningham and Sloper is particularly to be commended in this regard. In one study they looked at 24 children at the age of 42 weeks, comparing those who received intensive training with a control group. The intensive training group received coaching on object performance, imitation and span of attention for one hour daily. The control group just got general advice. They found there were positive short-term effects for the intensive training group, but this good effect was not sustained. The intensive training group were able in the short term to improve performance in specific tasks.

In any learning process there is a period when the learning process reaches a plateau while the child consolidates the achievement. During this period the child may be unreliable in repeatedly performing the task, and his learned performance appears to be unstable. For example, during potty training a child may have occasional 'accidents' for quite a while before becoming reliably dry.

Cunningham and Sloper showed in their study that the short-term benefit was due to improved stability of performance. There was, however, no evidence that the intensive training was actually altering the processes by which the task was learnt, or that it was accelerating development by reducing the effects of cumulative disability. If they had noticed gains in these latter two respects, longer-term benefit might have been expected.

Their work also showed that there is a positive correlation between the mother's secondary educational achievement and developmental attainment in the child with Down's syndrome; implying that genetic, as well as psychosocial, factors operate to determine outcome. Children with Down's syndrome also did better when they had families who loved and valued them for whom they were.

Nowadays a lot of pressure is put on parents, either from their own emotions or from the misguided energies of families or friends, to pursue intensive intervention programmes. The Doman Delacarto method is probably the best known, but it is just one of many. The American Academy of Pediatrics expressed concern over the Doman Delacarto programme in 1982. They found that the promotional methods often made it difficult for parents to refuse treatment; that the methods themselves were demanding, inflexible and stressful; that procedures put restrictions on age appropriate activities; and that, further, claims for dramatic improvement and cure were unsubstantiated. They commented that the treatment had no special merit, its claims were unproven and that the demands on families were so great that harm could result from its use.

Great caution certainly must be exercised before pursuing an intensive training programme as the child's disability becomes the focus and *raison d'être* for all the family, to the detriment of any brothers and sisters. When disability within a family assumes this importance it really has become a handicap.

The driving forces for families coerced in this way are very complex, but non-acceptance of the disability and unresolved grief are clearly important in some. Where non-acceptance does persist, and parents retain an urge to put 'their child right', then they must be helped to realise that intensive training and pseudo-scientific dietary regimens will not alter the end result. Money raised for expensive trips to an institute for human potential or for exotic vitamin concoctions might more usefully be donated to local services, which are so often in need of extra resources.

There is no doubt that parents may turn to alternative therapy if they perceive the professionals they have to deal with are taking a negative attitude. Doctors, in particular, are all too readily accused of shaking their heads where disability is concerned (see above). Equally, though, doctors and therapists must not fall into the trap of encouraging parents to believe they are 'healing'. There is a very fine line between presenting a therapy as something that will allow a person with Down's syndrome to develop their full potential and implying that the therapy will actually increase that potential to the point of cure. It is the magical belief that parents have in the healing powers of health professionals that take them off to institutes of therapy when they find themselves unable to adjust to the child's inherent rate of progress.

Community learning disability support

Most health authorities now have a community learning disability support team who are in a position to advise parents on various aspects of their child's life, and this will be the mainstay of 'therapy'. A child with Down's syndrome spends most hours of the week at home with parents. Where the parents are well adjusted to the problem and where the child is loved and valued, the quality of interaction between parents and the child will be good too. It is therefore the aim of therapists to offer advice on the sort of interaction that might be pursued to encourage the next developmental step.

Most district health authorities will have a disability register so that facilities for individual children can be coordinated. Access to facilities can be obtained by general practitioner referral to a local paediatrician or senior clinical medical officer (local community clinic doctor). The diagnostic services available at the local district general hospital will help define any medical problems, and specialist advice will complement the original counselling process.

Physio and occupational therapy

Much early development is dependent on motor skills. Children with Down's syndrome often have hypotonia (poor muscle tone), with poor muscle fixation at the shoulder and pelvis. Therapists can advise on the most suitable posturing, seating and play to develop these skills.

Speech therapy

Children with Down's syndrome often show language impairment over and above their general developmental disability. Initially, speech therapists can offer useful advice on the more severe speech problems, often in conjunction with the physiotherapist. Development of language concepts can be facilitated by the use of an alternative method of communication, such as Makaton, before speech develops. Some children with Down's syndrome reach school before speech has developed, but expressive language often improves at the same time as the acquisition of reading skills.

Speech therapy is a rare commodity in many local authorities. Nonetheless, parents should have confidence in themselves as teachers. What they do intuitively is often right!

Community nurse

The community nurse complements other members of the team by offering additional counselling, coordinating team members, giving out information and providing useful feedback. She may help families by introducing them to developmental checklists. Parents quickly forget what children learn to do in what order and a rough guide on what comes next in any area of development, along with advice about what to include in play to facilitate this, is welcome. There are many ways of achieving this. The approach may be unstructured, or quite well defined, as in the Portage scheme, where parents keep a continuing record of progress.

Educational and clinical psychologists

At some stage a more formal assessment of developmental attainment will be appropriate, undertaken by an educational psychologist. The purpose of this is two-fold; the planning of education, and the counselling of parents. Assessments allow members of the team to counsel parents on the range of ability their child is likely to have in future years, and from the age of 10 months or so assessments take on a predictive quality in this respect; from this age counsellors can say with at least 80 per cent certainty that a child will be mildly, moderately or severely learning impaired. Care must be taken not to confuse intellectual with social ability, remembering it is possible to be illiterate but to be quite able to care for oneself.

The psychologist is usually the best local person to provide parents with information on schools. The 1981 Education Act states that children with special needs are entitled to the benefits of education from the age of 2, although it must be acknowledged that not all education authorities have the resources to meet all children's needs. Usually, however, a good compromise can be reached between a family's hopes and expectations and what is actually available. Medical practitioners are asked to contribute to statements of special educational need, and that evidence is considered along with formal and semi-formal educational assessments (see Chapter 7). Very often it will be obvious where the child is best placed in school; at other times a trial placement must be made.

Clinical psychologists can offer useful child guidance if behavioural problems are causing stress within the family. The key aims are to help families identify the source of the child's frustration, and hopefully to overcome it. Consistency in approach is very important, not only between family members but also with staff at school, too.

At times behaviour patterns are more determined by the underlying brain problem itself rather than by the child's environment, particularly in the more severely disabled. In these circumstances behavioural therapy will not be wholly successful, and parents should be encouraged to seek respite care through local social services, and especially to do it without any feeling of shame or failure.

Social worker

Although limited resources may not allow the provision of a social worker for every community learning disability team, families are advised to have at least one consultation with the local department of social services. Two main questions should be addressed.

The first is to what allowances are the family entitled?

- At the age of 5 some families will be entitled to Mobility Allowance, available to those who have extreme difficulty in walking or who cannot walk at all. Previously this excluded many learning disabled children who could but did not always want to walk in the same direction as their parents! This was quite disabling where public transport was concerned but thankfully the situation has now changed. Claims are now assessed for children with learning disability.

- In April 1992 Attendance Allowance was replaced by Disability Living Allowance. This is available to all who have an illness or a disability and need help with personal care or getting around. An application for this allowance does not normally need a medical examination, nor is it means-tested and it helps many people who may previously have been turned down for either Mobility or Attendance Allowance. The allowance is available to all those under 66. To be able to apply for Diability Living Allowance people must normally have needed help for three months and must be likely to need help for a further six months or more. Clearly this applies to most people with Down's syndrome. In relation to personal care Disability Living Allowance covers the areas previously addressed by Attendance Allowance. It is designed to enable people to get help with daily living skills such as washing, dressing or using the toilet, help with preparing a cooked main meal (but only for the over 16s) or to provide someone to supervise activities. The welcome change to the mobility aspect of things is that it is now designed to accommodate those who are severely mentally impaired or with severe behavioural problems or those who can walk but need someone with them when out of doors. This will be a welcome change for many parents.
- Invalid care allowance will complement this in some cases, according to whether parents work and their income.
- Disability Working Allowance is available to those people who can work but whose illness or disability limits their earning capacity. This is a new benefit in the United Kingdom from April 1992 for those aged 16 and over. The allowance will not affect any monies received through an existing Attendance Allowance, Mobility Allowance or Disability Living Allowance. Full details of all allowances are available from local social services departments.

Social services should also be asked what provision they are making for the care of the adult disabled within their authority. There are two aspects to this:

- What plans for provision have actually been made?

● Is funding available?

Generally, good special educational facilities exist within authorities, but once children leave school, arrangements are far less satisfactory. Parents should be encouraged to press local authorities to draw up plans for such provision where they do not exist.

Meanwhile social workers can be very helpful in arranging respite care where it is needed. In childhood and teenage years this is often on a short-term basis initially. Local authorities have a number of small community homes for this purpose, but are increasingly recruiting families in the community to act as foster parents and to offer the children a 'home from home'. Parents are bound to feel reticent about this initially, although it is surprising how the children often relish the experience of 'weekends away'. The foster parents usually have children of their own, and it turns out to be something of an adventure for all concerned.

Summary

There is no evidence to suggest that either intensive intervention programmes or nutritional treatment alter the developmental potential of people with Down's syndrome in any important way. Parents often turn to these methods where they have found negative attitudes amongst the professionals they deal with or where they have unresolved grief and non-acceptance of the handicap. Changing the attitudes of doctors will take time, but unresolved parental grief and non-acceptance of the disability can both be helped with counselling.

Children with Down's syndrome spend most hours of the week at home with their parents. Where the parents are well adjusted to the problem, and where the child is loved and valued, the quality of interaction between parents and child will be naturally good. It should then be the aim of therapists to offer advice on the sort of interaction that is most likely to encourage the next developmental step.

Children with Down's syndrome are likely to do best where they are loved and valued for the individuals they are, and when they have good local professional advice to complement the loving encouragement of their parents.

11

The future

Whereas it is plain to see that huge advances have been made since Langdon Down wrote on the subject in the 1860s, there remains very much more to be achieved. The main advances are likely to be in the field of genetics and in our systems of education and social support for people with Down's syndrome.

The human genome project

The human genome is the total genetic information carried by the chromosomes in a human cell. The United States is investing a huge amount of money (83 million dollars in the year 1990–1 alone) to map it out, i.e. establish precisely which components of human metabolism are coded for at each site on each chromosome. This is a vast project and involves finding the exact location of all the 3 to 3.5 billion nucleotide base pairs (the chemical units that make up the information packages) on the human DNA molecule.

Methods of sequencing the base pairs are only just being developed, and it is not clear at what rate progress will be made, but this massive project, together with more modest ones in the United Kingdom, will result in us knowing exactly which biochemicals are coded for on the part of chromosome 21 that leads to the characteristics of Down's syndrome.

Unfortunately, the mere fact that one finds the exact location of some base pairs will not in itself unlock the secrets of life. However, it will give an initial insight into the interaction of biochemicals within the medium of the cell and how to manipulate those interactions to advantage.

Therapy

In practical terms it remains likely that the only way to study therapeutic intervention is by means of the randomised control trial. A long-term assessment of anti-oxidants such as vitamin E seems particularly appropriate, as anti-oxidants scavenge the biochemicals known as free radicals that appear to be implicated in many facets of disordered cell function in Down's syndrome. It can be foreseen that the logistics of such a trial, not to mention its ethics, will be problematical.

Meanwhile it is worth emphasising that there seems little point in blind blunderbussing with vitamin co-enzymes to drive on enzyme systems that are already overactive. It must also be acknowledged that, once more is known about chromosome 21 and its effect on metabolism, we may merely learn that it could never be put right and manipulated in a therapeutic way.

Attitude of doctors and health-care professionals

Doctors could in general improve their performance (and their public image) greatly by trying to be more positive about disability. If parents of a child with Down's syndrome are confronted by a positive attitude, they are more likely to take a positive view themselves.

Doctors therefore need to address their own feelings on the issue, to put themselves in the place of parents, and to ask themselves what it is they would want if they were in a similar position. Greater recognition of the psychological issues involved is likely to lead both to better care and to more emphasis being placed on counselling skills in the undergraduate medical curriculum.

Health screening programmes are generally well established in district health authorities. All children should have good assessment of sight and hearing. In Down's syndrome this needs to be extended universally to include other screening issues such as echocardiography at birth to identify those children with a heart defect. Through the early identification of the problem, all therapeutic choices are retained.

Educational changes

On the educational front, some parents of children with Down's syndrome have found themselves in difficulty since special schools for children with mild learning difficulties disappeared. Nowadays the choice is between placement in a school for children with moderate learning difficulties, or integration.

The integration experiment has been in the main under-resourced, and still relies heavily on the attitude of the headteachers involved. In the future it is to be hoped that each educational authority will develop policies and resources that will allow children with Down's syndrome a range of educational provision to suit individual needs, rather than fitting the child into an inflexible educational system.

Community services

Social services, in conjunction with local health authorities and voluntary organisations, need to develop plans for housing within their area. It is to be hoped that plans such as this will allow many the stated aim of 'having a place of their own'. The establishment of more opportunities for social integration is to be encouraged, while Gateway clubs and buddy systems have established value for all concerned.

Employers and staff in adult training centres need to recognise the work potential of many with Down's syndrome so that they can be placed in suitable employment. This will allow them a greater opportunity to develop their own potential and to live independently.

Final thoughts

1990, the year this book was first drafted, was described by some as the *anno mirabili*, the year of miracles, reference being made to the breakdown of international barriers, particularly in eastern Europe. For the first time in a long while the world was set for greater cooperation between national groups, always able to cooperate but never allowed to.

It is our hope that further development of the potential of people with Down's syndrome will allow the removal of the barriers put up against them by society. In this way friendships will develop and support systems flourish. We must always remember that one of the best determinants of developmental outcome is where children and adults with Down's syndrome find themselves in an environment where they are loved and valued for the individuals they are.

GLOSSARY

Adenoidectomy An operation to remove the adenoids which are lymph glands found in the upper part of the throat known as the naso-pharynx.

Alopecia Areas of baldness.

Alpha-fetoprotein Protein produced by the foetal liver which passes into the amniotic fluid and the maternal circulation where it is found in increased amounts in some foetal abnormalities or in lower than average amounts in Down's syndrome.

Alphatocopherol An antioxidant present in the diet.

Alzheimer's Disease A cause of pre-senile dementia where people lose their faculties at an early age which is common in Down's syndrome.

Amniocentesis The drawing off of some amniotic fluid contained in the sac which surrounds the growing foetus.

Amyloid A protein coded for on chromosome 21.

Aneuploidy Too many or too few chromosomes.

Anterior Commissure Connecting fibres between the two frontal lobes of the brain.

Antibodies Proteins produced by the body's immune system which help to neutralise infecting agents such as bacteria or viruses.

Anticholinesterase A drug which boosts the level of a neurotransmitter called acetyl-choline by preventing its breakdown.

Antioxidant Chemical substances such as vitamin E or alpha-tocopherol which inhibit oxidative processes in cells and thereby reduce the production of damaging free radicals.

Astigmatism An abnormality of the eye lens which distorts vision in more than one plane.

Atheroma A type of degeneration of the walls of arteries (main blood vessels) seen with advancing age.

Atlanto-axial instability The tendency for the first cervical vertebrum (the atlas) to slip on the second (the axis).

Atresia Failure in development of the hole through a hollow organ such as a bowel or blood vessel.

Atrium One of two low pressure chambers of the heart receiving blood from veins to pass on to the ventricles.

Autoantibodies Proteins produced by the body's immune system which have the potential to damage the body's own tissue.

Autoimmune disease A disorder of a variety of organs produced by the production of autoantibodies.

Beta-blockers Drugs which prevent the heart from being raced by the excitatory autonomic nervous system.

Biofeedback Mechanisms which control body functions with the use of sensors or receptors which are sensitive to the level of specific chemicals (and therefore switch off production for a while) or the level of nervous impulses as seen in the control of muscle tone.

Brainstem The long thin part of the brain on which the cerebral hemisphere and cerebellum lie. It contains the control centres for the muscles of the head and neck and vital bodily functions such as breathing.

Brushfield spots Speckling of the iris.

Canalisation Direction and organisation of a developmental process such as organ formation.

Cataract Opaque deposits in the eye lens causing difficulty with vision.

Cell A small discrete mass from which most living things are made, containing the protoplasm in which most of the chemical reactions on which life is dependent take place bounded by the cell-wall; in the centre is a nucleus containing the chromosomal material which directs the chemical processes.

Central nervous system The brain and spinal cord.

Centromere The spindle attachment of chromosomes.

Cerebellum One of the main motor control centres of the brain which receives and coordinates sensory information to modify motor output.

Chiasmata Connections between chromatids, visible during meiosis.

Chorionic villus biopsy Sampling of tissue from the sac containing the developing foetus, usually at about 12 weeks of gestational age.

Chromosome Thread-shaped body of which there are normally 23 pairs in the nucleus of each cell; made largely of DNA, they govern cell structure and function.

Chromotid One of two strands of a chromosome formed when the DNA material duplicates during mitosis or meiosis.

Coeliac disease Disease of the intestine leading to the malabsorption of nutrients, due to sensitivity to the gluten contained in cereals.

Coenzyme A substance, often a vitamin, playing an essential part in the reactions of enzyme systems; without being consumed in the process by being used in one step of the reaction but reconstituted by a later step.

Cranial nerve Peripheral nerve emerging from the brain to supply structures of the head.

Cutis marmorata Mottled skin rash taking up the pattern of the underlying small blood vessels.

Cyanosis Blueness of the tissues due either to poor blood supply or low oxygen concentration in the blood.

Cyclid guanine monophosphate The specific substance or substrate acted on by the enzyme guanylate cyclase; generating energy for cell wall function.

Cystathionine synthase An enzyme involved in the production of cystathionine which seems to protect against arteriosclerosis.

Dendrites Branching projections of nerve-cells which pass on and receive impulses from neighbouring nerves.

Dentition Arrangement of the teeth.

Differentiation Process of change in groups of cells as they form the different tissues and organs of the body both during foetal development and after injury.

Digoxin Drug to slow and increase the strength of the heart beat.

Disability The relatively poor function that results from a physical impairment, such as the poor vision that might result from cataracts.

DNA Deoxyribonucleic acid, a large number of nucleotides linked with a parallel strand by base-pairs and coiled in a helix. It is found mainly in the chromosomes where its power to reproduce some of the sequences of nucleotides leads to the production of proteins which make up cell structure and function.

DNA probe Chemical marker capable of identifying and locking on to a specific sequence of nucleotides.

Duodenum First part of the small intestine, leading from the stomach.

Dysembryogenesis Disorderly formation of an organ at an early stage in uterine life.

Dysfunction A disorder or function/malfunction.

Dyspraxia Difficulty in carrying out movements in a fluent way in spite of having a full capacity to move and with no weakness: poor coordination and sequencing of movement by the brain.

Dystrophic A disorder of the growth of an organ or system.

Echocardiography Imaging of the heart using ultra-sound.

Endocardial cushion A swelling of atrial canal tissue seen in the early embryo which acts as a seat for the mitral and tricuspid valves and from which the atrio-ventricular septum is formed.

Endocrine glands The glands which produce hormones.

Endoplasmic reticulum Complex system of paired membranes lying in the cytoplasm of the cell which contain many of the cell's enzyme systems.

Epicanthic folds The fold of skin seen at the inner nasal side of the eye.

Epilepsy A recurring abnormality of posture or tone, usually associated with an alteration of conscious level due to abnormal electrical discharge in the brain.

Folate Dietary substance which promotes normal growth in red blood and nerve-cells in particular.

Follicle-stimulating hormone Hormone produced by the pituitary gland which promotes the normal production of eggs and sperm.

Fore-brain The anterior, front division of the embyronic brain from which are formed the cerebral hemispheres, eyes, and part of the pituitary gland.

Free radical Oxygen-containing biochemical which can damage the energy production in cells if overproduced.

Gamete An egg or sperm.

Gene A unit of DNA on the chromosome which is responsible for the production of a specific protein.

Glossectomy Surgical removal of the tongue (usually partial).

Glycogen A biochemical made up of many glucose molecules: the form in which glucose is stored, particularly in the muscles and liver.

Glutathione peroxidase An enzyme which helps to control the production of free radicals.

Gonadotrophin The small group of hormones secreted by the pituitary gland which control the function of the ovaries and testicles.

Grommet Small, holed device which may be inserted into the ear-drum to effect drainage of fluid from the middle ear.

Guanylate-cyclase A membrane enzyme system which produces energy.

Handicap A disadvantage for an individual resulting from a disability and impairment which limits or prevents the fulfilment of a role or task. Poor coordination (the disability) due to brain structure (the impairment in Down's syndrome) may be a handicap when playing football but not when watching television.

Heteromorphism The variation of chromosomal structure which results from the crossing over of DNA from one to another at cell division.

Hyperextension Overextension.

Hyperkeratosis Scaliness of the skin due to an overproduction of keratin.

Hypermetropia Long-sightedness.

Hyperthyroid The clinical state resulting from an overactive thyroid gland.

Hyperploidy More than the usual number of chromosomes.

Hypoplasia Undergrowth of an organ.

Hypoploidy Less than the usual number of chromosomes.

Hypospadias Where the urethral opening (the exit hole for urine) falls short of the tip of the penis.

Hypothalamus Part of the brain which governs the function of the pituitary gland and the autonomic (automatic) nervous system.

Hypothyroid Clinical state associated with an underactive thyroid gland.

Hypotonia Where the resting activity in muscles (tone) is lower than usual.

Immune system/Immunity The body's defence system,

partly effected by lymphocytes (small white blood cells) produced in the thymus gland and partly by antibodies produced by lymphocytes originating elsewhere in the lymphatic system.

Impairment An abnormality of structure of an organ which may lead to a disability.

Interferon A complex protein with anti-viral properties.

Lacrimal gland The gland which produces tears.

Lecithin Fatty substance made up of glycerol, fatty acid, choline and phosphoric acid found in animal cells.

Leukaemia Cancerous overproduction of white blood cells.

Limbic system Part of the brain which includes the hypothalamus: it controls the autonomic (automatic) nervous system, the interpretation of smell and some aspects of learning.

Lipoperoxidation The involvement of fatty acids and cholesterol in oxidative metabolism (the adding of oxygen to their structure) which may disrupt cell structure and function if not well-controlled.

Luteinising hormone A gonadotrophin important in the control of ovulation.

Lymphocyte-functional antigen A substance which assists the binding of lymphocytes to foreign material (antigen).

Macroscopic Seen by the naked eye.

Malabsorption A deficiency in food contents being taken into the circulation due to poor function of the bowel wall.

Makaton Simple system of sign language.

Meiosis Two successive cell divisions which resemble mitosis but the chromosomes are only duplicated once resulting in this being the reduction division.

Membrane A layer of molecules which form a barrier.

Metabolism The chemical processes involved in living organisms which build up (anabolism) or break down (catabolism) organic biochemicals.

Methotrexate An anti-folate chemical used in the treatment of leukaemia.

Microscopic Seen only down the microscope; too small to be seen with the naked eye.

Microtubules The tiny filaments which make up the spindles at cell division.

Mitosis The usual process of cell division: the chromosomes duplicate and then there is a separation of these duplicates so that each daughter cell has the normal number of chromosomes.

Monoclonal antibody An antibody produced by a single cell line (clone) very specifically for a single antigen.

Monocyte Largest white cell involved in clearing the products of inflammation.

Mosaicism Where the body is made up of more than one population of cells, one with the normal number of chromosomes and the other with an abnormal number of chromosomes.

Myelography Special X-ray examination designed to outline the spinal cord.

Myopia Short-sightedness.

Myringotomy Opening up the ear-drum.

Nasolacrimal duct The tunnel through the tissues which joins the eye to the nose down which many tears pass.

Neuritic plaques One of the microscopic hallmarks of Alzheimer's disease seen in brain tissue.

Neurofibrillary tangles Another microscopic hallmark of Alzheimer's disease seen in brain tissue.

Neuropathy A disorder of the function of peripheral nerves which take information from the brain out from the spinal cord to the muscles.

Neurotransmitter A chemical released from a nerve ending which crosses the synapse to excite or inhibit activity in the adjoining nerve-cell.

Non-disjunction Failure of two similar (homologous chromosomes) to go to opposite poles at the first meiotic division so that one daughter cell has both of the pair and one has neither.

Nucleic acid Long-chain molecule such as DNA made up of a large number of nucleotides.

Nucleus The part of the cell which contains the chromosomes.

Odontoid process/peg A bony projection of the second cervical vertebrum (axis) which passes into a hole in the body of the first cervical verberum (atlas), thus forming the pivot for rotation of the head on the neck.

Oestriol An oestrogen hormone whose concentration rises during pregnancy when it is produced largely by the placenta.

Oncogene A cancer-susceptibility gene.

Ossicle One of the bones making up the sound conducting mechanism in the middle ear.

Paroxysmal Of sudden onset.

Phenotype The characteristic appearance or manifestation of a particular genetic make-up (the genotype).

Phosphofructokinase An enzyme involved in the metabolism of glucose.

Polyhydramnios Where too much amniotic fluid surrounds the foetus.

Positron-emission tomography Three-dimensional imaging of the brain to display specific biochemical functions by using radio-active isotopes.

Primitive reflexes Involuntary, reflex patterns of movement seen in the developing foetus or young infant, usually controlled at spinal or brain-stem level, which disappear in the first few months of life as more complex patterns of movement emerge.

Proteinaceous Largely made up of protein.

Psychosis Disorder of the mind or mental illness which interferes with a person's ability to make sense of the world and what is seen, heard or felt.

Purines Biochemicals including adenine and guanine which are some of the base-building blocks which make up DNA.

Pyridoxal-5-phosphate Related to vitamin B6 this plays an important part in brain metabolism.

Pyrimidines Biochemicals including thymine and cytosine which are some of the base-building blocks which make up DNA.

Ritalin An addictive drug (other name methylphenidate) which has been used in the control of hyperactive behaviour.

Schilling test A test to evaluate the absorption of vitamin B12.

Seborrhoeic dermatatis An inflammatory, scaling condition of hairy areas of skin which have a lot of sebaceous glands.

Selenium A trace element essential for a number of enzyme systems.

Septum Partition or wall.

Serotonin Also known as 5-hydroxytryptamine this is an important neurotransmitter.

Serum Blood plasma minus its clotting constituents.

Spermatogenesis The normal process of sperm production by the testicle.

Spinal cord The part of the central nervous system which lies in the backbone; the nerve fibres are taking motor information down to and transmitting sensory information up from each segmental level of the body.

Somatomedin An important growth hormone produced by the pituitary gland.

Spindle Body formed in cells during mitosis and meiosis which takes part in the distribution of the chromatids to the two daughter nuclei.

Stenosis Abnormal narrowing of a hollow structure such as a blood vessel or bowel.

Superoxide dismutase Enzyme involved in the metabolism of binding oxygen to biochemicals: the result is the production of free radicals.

T-cell Thymus-dependent lymphocytes involved in cell-mediated body defences.

Testosterone The principal male sex-steroid hormone.

Thymus gland A primary lymphoid organ in the upper part of the chest where T-cells mature.

Thyroid An endocrine gland in the neck which produces hormones which control growth and the rate of body metabolism.

Thyroxine Hormone produced by the thyroid gland.

Trace element A substance which must be available to the body in very small amounts to ensure good health: they act as constituents in enzyme systems e.g. copper, molybdenum, selenium and so on.

Translocation Transfer of part of a chromosome onto a different part of a chromosome of the same type (homologous) or different (non-homologous) type.

Trial A method of working out the effectiveness of a treatment (a drug or perhaps a method of physiotherapy). The effect of the treatment is measured in a study group and compared to a control group of subjects who had no treatment or perhaps a long-established method of treatment. Placebos are often used in the control group. Trials may be double-blind where neither doctor nor subject know whether the treatment is drug or placebo (a record of treatment usually being kept by a third person such as a pharmacist).

Trimester One of three, three-month periods which make up pregnancy in humans.

Tri-iodothyronine A hormone produced by the thyroid gland.

Trisomy Describes a nucleus containing three of one type of chromosome instead of the usual two.

Tympanic membrane The ear-drum.

Tympanosclerosis Distortion of the ear-drum with scar-tissue.

Ventricle A chamber. There are two in the heart which act as the muscular pumping chambers. There are four in the brain through which and in which the cerebro-spinal fluid flows.

Vertibrum One of the bones making up the spinal column, through which passes the spinal cord.

Vitamins Substances which are vital for normal body metabolism: usually acting as co-enzymes ensuring the smooth and fast running of enzyme-systems.

Vitiligo Skin condition where areas of the skin contain no pigment, at times associated with autoimmune disease elsewhere in the body.

Zygoma The cheek bone.

ABOUT THE DOWN'S SYNDROME ASSOCIATION

As a result of parents wanting the best for their children with Down's syndrome, voluntary organisations have been formed which work in partnership with the professionals. One such organisation is the Down's Syndrome Association; founded in 1970 as the Down's Babies Association, it grew with its original families to become the Down's Children's Association in 1973, and finally the Down's Syndrome Association in 1986. The Down's Syndrome Association is now the leading UK organisation for children and adults with Down's syndrome, for their families and for the professionals who work with them.

The Association aims:

- To create and develop the conditions that will enable people with Down's syndrome to become people with prospects.
- To give support to parents through individuals and local groups, particularly at the crucial time around birth.
- To promote the care, nurture and education of people with Down's syndrome, especially in the early years of life.
- To increase both public awareness and understanding of the nature of Down's syndrome, and the capacity of people with Down's syndrome to lead rewarding and full lives.
- To promote research into the care, nurture and education of people with Down's Syndrome, and to publicise such research.

The DSA provides direct help to members and others:

- By providing immediate support and assistance for new parents via the 24-hour helpline and the network of parents who already have a child with Down's syndrome.
- By helping families and professionals set up local self-help

groups so that they can share their problems and successes.

- By giving up-to-date objective information and advice on a wide range of subjects, from early feeding problems, education, adolescence, to life after school.

- By maintaining a resource centre in London with a range of books, literature, videos and other specialist publications.

- By producing a national newsletter, available to all members of the DSA, containing news, tips and ideas on all matters relating to Down's syndrome, up-to-date information and research findings.

USEFUL ADDRESSES

Support organisations

Afasic (Association for All Speech Impaired Children)
347 Central Markets, Smithfields Lane,
London, EC1A 9HN.
Tel: 0171 236 3632

Ace (Advisory Centre for Education)
1 Aberdeen Studios, 22–24 Highbury Grove, London, N5.
Tel: 0171 354 8321

Children's Legal Centre
University of Essex,
Wivenhoe Park, Colchester, Essex, CO4 3SQ.
Tel: 01206 873820

Contact a Family
170 Tottenham Court Road, London, W1P 0HA.
Tel: 0171 383 3555

Down's Syndrome Association
155 Mitcham Road, London, SW17 9PG.
Tel: 0181 682 4001

IPSEA (Independent Panel for Special Education Advice)
22 Warren Hill Road, Woodbridge,
Suffolk, JP12 4DU.
Tel: 01394 382814

CSIE (Centre for Studies on Inclusive Education)
1 Redland Close, Elm Lane,
Redland, Bristol, BS6 6UE.
Tel: 0117 923 8450

Mencap
117–123 Golden Lane, London, EC1Y 0RT.
Tel: 0171 454 0454

National Deaf Children's Society
15 Dufferin Street, London, EC1V 8PD.
Voice & Minicom: 0171 250 0123

Rathbone Society
1st Floor, Excalibur Building, 77 Whitworth Street,
Manchester, M1 6EZ.
Tel: 0161 236 5358
This organisation produces literature helpful when seeking to
make a parental contribution to the statement.

SCOPE (Campaigns and Parliamentaty Dept.)
16 Fitzroy Square, London, W1P 6LP.
Tel: 0171 387 9571

Speakeasy (The Association of Speech Impaired)
34 Newark Street, London, E1 2AA.
Tel: 0171 377 7177

Council for Disabled Children
(Coordinating body)
8 Wakely Street, London, EC1V 7QE.
Tel: 0171 843 6000

**The Law Society's Group for the Welfare of People with a
Mental Handicap**
The Smokery, Greenhill's Rents, Cowcross Street, London,
EC1M 6BN.
Tel: 0171 251 5700

The Law Society's Mental Health Sub-Committee
The Law Society's Hall, 113 Chancery Lane,
London, WC2A 1PL.
Tel: 0171 252 1222

Disability Law Service (formerly Network)
Room 241, 2nd Floor, 49–51 Bedford Row,
London, WC1R 4LR.
Tel: 0171 831 8031

The Ravenswood Foundation
17 Highfield Road, Golders Green, London, NW11 9DZ.
Tel: 0181 458 3282

Department of Social Security
The Adelphi, 1–11 John Adam Street, London, WC2N 6HT.
Tel: 0171 962 8000

Portage

Nfer
Nelson Danille House, 2 Oxford Road East, Windsor, Berks, SL4 1DF.

Parent groups

Network 81
1–7 Woodfield Terrace, Stansted, Essex, CM24 8AJ.
Tel: 01279 647415
This is a growing national network of support groups run by and for parents whose children have disabilities or learning difficulties.

Case (Campaign for State Education)
Information from: 158 Durham Road, London, SW20 0DG.
Tel: 0181 844 8206

Professional help

Sarah Duffen Centre
Belmont Street, Southsea, PO5 1NA.
Sue Buckley – Director/Psychologist
Tel: 01705 824261
This trust provides weekends for parents with opportunities to discuss problems with professionals.

Advice on heart problems

The Down's Heart Group
17 Cantilupe Close, Eaton Bray, Dunstable, Beds, LU6 2EA.
Tel: 01525 2203

Home Farm Trust

Merchants House North, Wapping Road, Bristol, BS1 4RW.
Tel: 01272 273746
Residential home for adults with a learning disability.

FURTHER READING

The Development of Language and Reading Skills in Children with Down's Syndrome. Buckley, S., Emslie, M., Haslegrave, G. and LePrevost, P. Portsmouth Polytechnic, 1986.

Current Approaches to Down's Syndrome, Eds. Lane, D., Sratford, B. Holt, Rinehart and Winston, 1985.

Down's Syndrome – An Introduction for Parents. Dunningham, Cliff. Souvenir Press, 1990.
Probably the most comprehensive and readable book on Down's syndrome ever written. £8.95 (B).

Down's Syndrome: The Facts. Selikowitz, Mark. Oxford University Press, 1990.
A good guide with lots of useful and basic information. £6.99 (B).

Helping your Handicapped Baby. Cunningham, Cliff and Sloper, P. Souvenir Press, 1978.
Gives programmes for teaching and stimulating a handicapped child through the first year. Temporarily out of print.

After I'm Gone – What will Happen to my Handicapped Child? Sanctuary, Gerald. Souvenir Press, 1991.
A splendid, practical account of possibilities for care etc. £8.95 (B).

Children with Special Needs. Woolfson, Richard. Faber & Faber, 1991.
A general guide for parents and carers of a child with special needs.

Down's Syndrome – Moving Through Life. Eds. Burns, Yvonne and Gunn, Pat. Chapman & Hall, 1993.
Suggests activities that will encourage effective patterns of movement through the life span, everything from learning to suck and starting to move around, in the baby, right up to keeping fit in the adult. Written for parents and professionals.

Down's Syndrome: Children Growing Up – A Longitudinal

Perspective. Carr, Janet. Cambridge University Press, 1995.
A unique collection of data spanning the first 21 years of a cohort of people with Down's syndrome. A wide range of factors are studied from behaviour and discipline, self care and independence, through to effects on the family and provision of services.

Working Together with Handicapped Children. Griffiths, M. and Russell, P. Souvenir Press, 1985.
Reinforces to professionals the value of working in partnership with parents. £5.95 (B).

Behaviour Problems in Handicapped Children. Jones, Malcolm. Souvenir Press, 1983.
The Beech Tree House approach. £5.95 (B).

Let Me Speak. Jeffree and McConkey. Souvenir Press, 1991.
A good guide with helpful exercises, ideas etc. £5.99 (B).

Let's Talk. McConkey and Price. Souvenir Press, 1986.
A guide to learning language in everyday settings. £5.95 (B).

Mummy Why have I got Down's Syndrome? Philps, Caroline. Lion Press, 1991.
A moving account of a mother's reactions to having a child with Down's syndrome. £3.50 (B).

Your Name is Olga. Espinas, Josep. Unwin Hyam, 1989.
A splendid interchange of letters between an author and his daughter with Down's syndrome. £5.95 (B).

Let Me Play. Jeffree and McConkey. Souvenir Press, 1988.
Play ideas, advice and information. £6.95 (B).

Easy to Make Toys for your Handicapped Child. Caston, Don. Souvenir Press, 1983.
Some interesting projects. £5.95 (B).

Cookery for Handicapped People. Hargreaves, Jim. Souvenir Press, 1986.
A fascinating collection of ideas. £8.95 (B).

My Class Enjoys Cooking. Thomson, Ruth and Murray, Maggie. Franklin Watts, 1987.
The authors meet class members including Phillip Jones, a boy with Down's syndrome. £5.95 (B).

Communication Skills in Children with Down's Syndrome: A Guide for Parents. Kumin, Libby. Woodbine House, 1995.
Covers early communication skills, the development of language, how to improve articulation, the role of signing and reading. Sound practical advice given, though resources listed are often not available outside the USA.

Managing Problem Behaviours – A Practical Guide for Parents and Teachers of Young Children with Special Needs. Dodd, Susan. Maclennan & Petty, 1994.
Offers a range of easy to follow tips and strategies to help solve most behaviour problems in young children.

My Cook Book. Marshall, Rosamund. BILD, 1993.
Recipes and kitchen tips for people who may have difficulty reading a traditional cookery book. Designed for the individual at home and the teacher and pupils at school.

Sixteen and Then What. McCormack, Andrina. Hodder and Stoughton, 1989.
Contributes much to the understanding of young adults with a learning disability. £5.25 (B).

Mental Handicap and Sexuality. Craft, Ann. Costello, 1989.
A sensitive, caring approach to every issue surrounding this subject. £12.95 (B).

Growing Up. Meredith, Susan. Usborne Books, 1985.
A useful guide to adolescence, body changes and sex which has a readable, non-threatening text and good illustrations. £3.95 (B).

The Adolescent with Down's Syndrome. Buckley and Sacks. Portsmouth Down's Syndrome Trust, 1987.
A clear and illuminating account of life for the teenager and for the family. £6.95 (B).

After Age 16 What Next? Cowen, Alison. Family Fund, 1993.
Information on services and benefits for young people with disabilities. Free from the Family Fund to people with a disability and their families.

Shared Feelings. Maksym, Diane. G Allan Roeher Institute, 1990.
A parent guide to education about relationships and sexuality for children, adolescents and adults with learning disabilities.

Mental Handicap & Sexuality: Issues and Perspectives. Craft, Ann. Costello Publishers Ltd.
Covers perceptions of sexuality, emotional needs, sex education programmes, parents' views and the experiences of relationships by people with learning disabilities.

INDEX